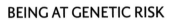

BEING AT GENETIC RISK

RSA·STR

THE **RSA** SERIES IN TRANSDISCIPLINARY **RHETORIC**

The *RSA Series in Transdisciplinary Rhetoric* is a collaboration with the Rhetoric Society of America to publish innovative and rigorously argued scholarship on the tremendous disciplinary breadth of rhetoric. Books in the series take a variety of approaches, including theoretical, historical, interpretive, critical, or ethnographic, and examine rhetorical action in a way that appeals, first, to scholars in communication studies and English or writing, and, second, to at least one other discipline or subject area.

Kelly Pender

BEING AT
GENETIC RISK

Toward a Rhetoric of Care

THE PENNSYLVANIA STATE UNIVERSITY PRESS
UNIVERSITY PARK, PENNSYLVANIA

Library of Congress Cataloging-in-Publication Data

Names: Pender, Kelly, 1974– author.
Title: Being at genetic risk : toward a rhetoric of care / Kelly
     Pender.
Other titles: RSA series in transdisciplinary rhetoric.
Description: University Park, Pennsylvania : The Pennsylvania
     State University Press, [2018] | Series: The RSA series in
     transdisciplinary rhetoric | Includes bibliographical
     references and index.
Summary: "Advocates a conversation around the genetic risk
     for breast and ovarian cancers that focuses less on choice
     and more on care. Offers a new set of conceptual starting
     points for understanding what is at stake with a BRCA
     diagnosis and what the focus on choice obstructs from
     view"—Provided by publisher.
Identifiers: LCCN 2018030803 | ISBN 9780271082103 (cloth :
     alk. paper)
Subjects: LCSH: BRCA genes. | Breast—Cancer—Patients—
     Medical care. | Ovaries—Cancer—Patients—Medical care. |
     Genetic screening. | Rhetoric.
Classification: LCC RC268.44.B73 P46 2018 |
     DDC 616.99/449—dc23
LC record available at https://lccn.loc.gov/2018030803

A portion of chapter 4 previously appeared as: Kelly Pender,
"Somatic Individuality in Context, a Comparative Case Study,"
Public Understanding of Science 27, no. 3 (2018): 338–51, first
published online, November 21, 2016. Copyright © 2016 Kelly
Pender. Reprinted by permission of Sage Publications.

The Pennsylvania State University Press is a member of the
Association of University Presses.

For JMV and EJV

Contents

Acknowledgments

Above everyone else, I want to thank the BRCA+ women who shared with me their experiences of living with genetic risk of breast and ovarian cancers. I am grateful for their openness about the practical details of those experiences, as I would not have been able to write this book without them. Nor would I have been able to write this book without the support of my colleagues in the English Department at Virginia Tech and beyond. Not long after I came to Virginia Tech in 2006, my research interests began shifting toward medical rhetoric, and no one did more to make that a productive shift than Karen Kopelson and Bernice Hausman. Since graduate school, Karen has been a trusted reader and cherished friend, and I thank her for providing early feedback that helped this book to take shape. Through her support, advice, reading recommendations, and our countless conversations, Bernice has also helped this book take shape, and I hope she knows how very much I appreciate her as both a friend and mentor. I also greatly appreciate the support of my colleague Carlos Evia, whose steadfast friendship has made every day at work a better day. I am grateful that he and his family, Jane and Sofia, are part of my life and the life of my family. Likewise, I want to acknowledge Katy Powell, her husband Joe, and their son Henry, the three people who have been our Blacksburg family for over a decade now. Support from English Department colleagues has also come from Gena Chandler-Smith, Carolyn Rude, Nancy Metz, Ginney Fowler, Julie Mengert, Patty Norris, Jennifer Mooney, Eve Trager, and Bridget Szerszynski. I am lucky to work in a place where people care about and for each other in the ways that these co-workers do.

I also want to thank graduate students, past and present, for their support and encouragement throughout this project. Amy Reed and Heidi Lawrence have helped me think through various parts of this work, and I am happy to count them as close colleagues. The students in my spring 2017 Theories of Written Communication class also helped me work through parts of this book, as we spent many hours of class discussing what new materialism did and did not bring to scholarship in rhetoric and writing studies. In particular, I want to thank Brooke Covington, Alexis Priestley, Katie Randall, Kelly Scarff, and

Katie Garahan for making those conversations so productive. I'd also like to thank a former Virginia Tech MFA student, Ana-Christina Acosta Gaspar de Alba, for her careful work helping me format and prepare the manuscript.

If I have a debt to those I've taught, then I also have one to those who taught me, especially Janice Lauer and Thomas Rickert. As any student of Janice's will tell you, her impact came not just through what she taught but also (and more so) through her expectations for doing good work. I'm not saying I've lived up to those expectations here, but they still guide me as a teacher and as a researcher, and so any success I have is, in part, the result of Janice's influence. Thomas has also been an important influence, both directly as a teacher and a friend and indirectly through his work, from which I have learned a great deal.

Kendra Boileau, editor-in-chief at Penn State University Press, has been a great help with this project, as have the editors for the RSA Series in Transdisciplinary Rhetoric, Leah Ceccarelli and Michael Bernard-Donals. I appreciate their support, feedback, and patience throughout the long process of writing this book. I also greatly appreciate the feedback of my two reviewers, Jodi Nicotra and Celeste Condit, both of whom provided generous and helpful feedback. I need to especially thank Celeste Condit, who has impacted this book not only as a reviewer who provided spot-on suggestions for revisions but also as a scholar whose work on rhetoric and genetics has been indispensible to my thinking on those two subjects.

A final thanks goes to my husband, Matthew Vollmer, and our son, Elijah Vollmer. In 2011, when Elijah was nine years old, I thanked him in a different book for being the perfect antidote for my preoccupation with work. This is still the case in 2018, and though the particular type of distraction he provides has changed, I remain so grateful for him and the way he keeps everything in perspective for me. To say that I am also grateful for Matthew is a tremendous understatement, as I could not have done this without his love, his support, and the life we've built together over the past eighteen years.

Introduction

In her 2008 book, *The Logic of Care: Health and the Problem of Patient Choice*, Annemarie Mol laments the fact that over the past several decades the bioethical principle of autonomy and its corollary "logic of choice" have played such a dominant role in defining what counts as good medicine. While certainly not advocating a return to the coercive practices of medicine's past, Mol argues that autonomy and choice are poor ideals for people who are sick. Shaped by a false binary between a paternalistic paradigm in which doctors make all decisions and a civic/consumerist one in which patients can have what they want, this logic values and, indeed, valorizes a type of freedom that is beyond the reach of most patients. That is, the logic of choice promotes the image of rational decision makers who, by weighing various options and exercising their purchasing power, can take control of their health. Yet the reality, Mol argues, is that people who are sick are neither in control nor ever truly free to choose (40–41).

Since the early days of the Human Genome Project (HGP), scholars in the social sciences and humanities have been arguing that those at genetic risk of disease face the same predicament. In other words, they have been arguing that choice is as poor an ideal for those whose genes predispose them to a disease as it is for those who have a disease. Typically, these arguments have focused on critique, aiming to expose the means by which logics and rhetorics of choice have allowed those at genetic risk to believe that they have freely chosen what they were, in fact, compelled to choose.

While I recognize the historical necessity of such critique, I worry, as Mol does, that it rarely produces the emancipatory effects at which it aims. Patients often experience a lack of choice, but are we always to assume that this lack of choice calls for emancipation? Are we to assume, in other words, that when patients experience a lack of freedom, it is because they have been submitted to the force of an institutional or ideological authority? In Mol's view, such an assumption overlooks the fact that people who are sick are not free because their bodies—which, in some fashion or another, don't function properly—require that they engage in care practices in order to live a good life. This requirement is not one from which patients can be liberated. Thus, Mol argues that in order to improve health care, we must turn our attention toward these care practices, putting the rationales that they embody into words so as to offer an alternative to the logic of choice rather than another critique of it. She terms this alternative, appropriately enough, *a logic of care*.

In brief, the primary aim of *Being at Genetic Risk: Toward a Rhetoric of Care* is to apply Mol's work within the context of genetic risk, specifically genetic risk for breast and ovarian cancers due to a BRCA mutation.[1] Thus, while my argument begins with a problem that has been identified by many before me (the fact that choice is a poor ideal for the genetically at risk), it responds to this problem differently, extending Mol's work to demonstrate that for those at genetic risk, a lack of freedom does not necessarily require (or cannot always be remedied by) emancipation. Much of what the genetically at risk say and do, I maintain, escapes the questions of choice and empowerment that have dominated the discourses of genetic medicine and its critics for more than two decades. Thus, we need an alternative way of thinking and talking about their experience. However, rather than conceiving of this alternative as a logic of care, as Mol did, I have conceived of it as a rhetoric of care or, more specifically, as a set of conceptual starting places, or topoi, that can be used to foster a rhetoric of care by highlighting those elements of being at risk that choice (whether it is envisioned as an ethical ideal, an ideological illusion, or a governmental strategy) obstructs from view. Importantly, the primary goal of bringing these other elements into view is not to better represent the experience of being at genetic risk of breast and ovarian cancers. Topoi are better understood as tools than as explanations or representations, and while the specific topoi that I offer here are based on my analysis of various discourses surrounding BRCA risk,[2] they are not meant first and foremost to be a means of explaining those discourses. Rather, these topoi, like all good heuristics, are designed to help us invent and intervene, to move our minds out of their "habitual grooves," as Richard Young once put it, in order to see and act anew (Young 59).

While the primary aim of this book is, indeed, to help us think differently about the experience of being at risk of breast and ovarian cancers, it also seeks to contribute to our understanding of rhetoric. It does this by demonstrating the role that rhetorical invention understood as a productive art, or *techne*, can play in rhetoric of science, technology, and medicine (RSTM) scholarship.

Invention as a productive art has been a major concern in composition and communication pedagogy, but it has had little impact in rhetorical studies of discourse. Typically, when we study the rhetoric of something—a particular discipline, organization, public, or group, for instance—we want to know how that rhetoric performs, that is, how it creates knowledge, constitutes audiences and subjects, secures adherence, selects and deflects realities, and so on. But over the past ten years or so, the introduction and incorporation of new materialist theory into the humanities and social sciences has raised questions about the hermeneutic bent of this type of work, creating, in the process, an exigence for rethinking the role that invention can play as a mode of critical engagement in our field. Evidence of that rethinking is clear in publications like the 2013 issue of *POROI*, the purpose of which was "to stimulate conversation about the inventional resources" for scholarship in RSTM (Keranen 1), as well as in more recent work like Walsh and Boyle's 2017 *Topologies as Techniques for a Post-Critical Rhetoric*, a collection of essays that turn to various notions and practices of topology in order to provide inventive responses to the kinds of wicked problems that more traditional forms of critique have been unable to solve.

Being at Genetic Risk provides further evidence of this rethinking of invention, as it draws on the work of rhetoricians like Richard McKeon, Janet Atwill, and John Muckelbauer in order to demonstrate *not* how rhetoric performs in the biosocial discourses surrounding BRCA risk but instead how that rhetoric can be *made to perform* (Muckelbauer, *The Future of Invention* 43). As I will elaborate later, there is no hard-and-fast line between these two activities, and certainly I spend plenty of time in this book explaining how rhetoric performs, but I believe that within those explanations we can orient toward invention, as Muckelbauer puts it, and through that orientation find ways of intervening without demystifying. In arguing for this orientation, my goal is not to privilege invention over hermeneutics as much as it is to move away from a specific kind of hermeneutics that operates within critique, namely a hermeneutics of suspicion.[3] Ultimately I believe that we can interpret with the aim of invention, and that we can interpret with the aim of critique or demystification. Rhetorical studies of genetic risk have historically aimed for this latter set of goals, but as those goals have themselves become suspect, we find ourselves in need of new ways of engaging the discourses that matter to us. It is by responding to this need that *Being at Genetic Risk* seeks to contribute to our understanding of rhetoric.

Getting the Object Wrong

My decision to respond to the problem of choice by trying to foster a rhetoric of care is the product of many factors, not the least of which is how convincingly Mol illustrates and calls for such a response in *The Logic of Care*. But my thinking about the problem of choice in relation to genetic risk began taking shape before I read Mol's book. To be specific, the arguments I present here began to form in 2008, the year I tested negative for a BRCA mutation but was warned by the oncologist who was treating me not to assume that I was off the hook. I had a family history of breast cancer, but that history didn't look like a BRCA family history, and without being able to test my mother, who had died in 1989, my negative result didn't mean a whole lot. In other words, the message from my doctor was *be vigilant*, because probably there was some other kind of mutation floating around in my family, maybe one of unknown significance, and I should not assume that since it wasn't on one of the two BRCA genes, that it wouldn't affect me.

Although I was not vigilant in the way my doctor advised (meaning I did not embark on the recommended cancer-screening regimen or have risk-reducing surgery), I did become concerned enough to begin searching for information about genetic susceptibility to breast cancer. Among other places, that search led me to the website of an organization called FORCE, which stands for Facing Our Risk of Cancer Empowered. As the largest nonprofit organization for women and men[4] who have or are at risk of having hereditary breast and ovarian cancers, FORCE is the epicenter of the biosocial universe surrounding BRCA risk. *Biosocial* is a term that I will use often in this book, as it names the primary type of discourse on which I have focused this study: that which is produced by or about people with inherited predispositions to disease in order to help them manage the medical, social, and psychological issues associated with their predisposition. The term comes from the work of anthropologist Paul Rabinow, who predicted that various forms of "biosociality" would emerge as a result of the HGP. Writing in 1992, well before the appearance of widely available genetic tests, Rabinow argued that as research on the human genome progressed, groups of people would come to know themselves according to the "new truths" produced by genetic medicine, and by "new truths" Rabinow didn't mean knowledge about "some hypothetical gene for aggression or altruism" (244). To the contrary, he wrote, groups will form around specific alterations in the four nucleotides that make up human DNA, and these groups "will have medical specialists, laboratories, narratives, traditions, and a heavy panoply of pastoral keepers to help them experience, share, intervene in, and 'understand' their fate" (244). This vision of the future is clearly borne out by the FORCE website, whose users often refer to themselves as carriers of particular genetic mutations that confer particular types of cancer risk, for instance as "another 187delAG" or a member of the "8525delCs." But more important than the organization's association with this type of molecularized identity (at least to me) are the ways in which it tries to help BRCA+ women "experience, share, intervene in, and 'understand' their fate." In addition to providing information about topics ranging from cancer genetics and clinical trials to strategies for managing risk and choosing physicians, FORCE raises money for research, holds an annual conference, publishes a newsletter and brochures, offers a webinar series, advocates for (or against) policies that affect its members, and provides online forums through which users can seek advice and share their experiences. Its founder, Sue Friedman, is also a co-author of one of the most popular guidebooks about BRCA risk, *Confronting Hereditary Breast and Ovarian Cancer*. Thus, while FORCE is by no means alone in the biosocial universe of BRCA risk, with its website receiving over one million hits and over thirty thousand visits per month, it does stand at the center of that universe, acting as precisely the kind of "pastoral keeper" that Rabinow envisioned.

As Nikolas Rose points out in *The Politics of Life Itself*, "pastoral" in this context is not synonymous with a kind of "Christian pastorship" where the sheep must follow the shepherd but instead draws on the ethical principles of informed consent, autonomy, and choice to suggest a more dynamic and egalitarian relationship between those who counsel and the counseled (74, 29). As Rose also notes, though, in our "age of biological prudence" these ethical principles blur the line between coercion and consent, as they are "translated into microtechnologies for the management of communication and information that are inescapably normative and directional" (29). In other words, "pastoral keepers" like FORCE rely on a rhetoric of choice to provide information that inevitably promotes *certain* choices, and while I couldn't deny that as someone in need of counseling I found that information helpful, I also couldn't deny that I was bothered by its subtly coercive power. Thus, my interest in the site and the broader issues it represented took an academic turn, as I began contemplating and, indeed, critiquing these "microtechnologies." I was particularly uneasy with the way that FORCE and similar biosocial organizations seemed to accept and even valorize the "at risk" identity, using the term *previvor* to describe those who had "survived" their risk of breast and ovarian cancers. Further reading on the political and social functions of genetic risk corroborated my uneasiness with this term and the website in general, demonstrating through studies of various scientific, public, and mass media discourses that genetic medicine "geneticized" illness and identity, leading those labeled "at risk" to make compulsory medical choices that had severe iatrogenic side effects and, in the case of BRCA risk, often reinforced heterosexist gender norms. As I continued reading over the next year, however, the source of my unease shifted. A great deal of the scholarship on genetic risk seemed to assume that those who made decisions based on this "at risk" identity did so because they had been tricked. Thus, the implication was that they would choose differently, or at least more freely, if they knew better, that is, if they knew how and by what forces they had been tricked. Eventually, this implication (and the assumption it is based on) became a greater source of unease—and thus a more compelling exigence—than the problems represented by the site itself. In other words, eventually I came to believe that if rhetorics of choice in the new genetics were the problem, then critiques of those rhetorics could no longer be the default solution.

That I came to this conclusion is perhaps unsurprising. The limitations of critique are well known, as we have seen time and again that our efforts to reveal the oppressive machinations hiding behind or within some kind of rhetorical construction do not produce the positive social change we envision. In rhetoric studies, explanations of this failure have typically focused on the subject, on how we have misunderstood its relationship to ideology, for instance, or not fully grasped the ways in which it is a material production rather than just a discursive effect. Psychoanalytic theory has been instrumental in such arguments, allowing scholars like Marshall Alcorn and Thomas Rickert to demonstrate that because ideological commitments play a positive role in subject formation, they cannot simply be dissolved through a rational process of critique in which one discourse is replaced by another.[5] Others have turned to the work of philosopher Peter Sloterdijk, using his notion of enlightened false consciousness to argue that critique fails because it makes us cynics, that is, subjects who know that in our activity we are following an illusion, but who persist in doing it anyway (Sloterdijk). This was Victor Vitanza's argument in his 1999 address to the Research Network Forum at CCCC, where he challenged proponents of cultural studies and critical pedagogies to consider (and indeed study) the possibility that efforts to eliminate racist, sexist, classist, and consumerist behaviors among students were actually making them more cynical practitioners of those behaviors (700). In communication, Ronald Walter Greene has repeatedly raised questions about the efficacy of critique, identifying in both the critical rhetoric and constitutive rhetoric traditions a tendency to define rhetorical subjectivity as the "meaning effect" of the discursive processes inherent in texts ("Rhetorical Materialism" 50). Drawing primarily on Foucault's later work, Greene argued that such a view is inadequate because it privileges a bipolar model of power and a logic of representation, thus inhibiting our ability to understand rhetoric and the kinds of subjectivity it gives rise to in the more materialist terms of governing apparatuses and technologies of production ("Another Materialist" 24).

These and other efforts to locate the limitations of critique in inadequate conceptions of subjectivity clearly have a great deal of explanatory power, and for someone hoping to show why critiques of choice were not achieving the emancipatory effects we hoped for, there is no doubt that they would have been a valuable resource. But by the time I began working on this project, I, like so many others in our field, had become convinced that responding more effectively to the problems that matter to us would depend on our ability and willingness to begin giving objects their due, learning how to treat them as matters of concern rather than matters of fact, as Bruno Latour has taught us to put it. This phrase, "giving objects their due," has become a favorite piece of shorthand for signaling one's affiliation with the ontological turn that has galvanized work in the social sciences and humanities over the past several years. Richard Marback was the first in rhetoric studies to use it, arguing in his 2008 essay about the Joe Louis monument in Detroit that because objects are not just "featureless repositories of consequential responses," we must learn how to give them their due, recognizing that in our encounters with them, they "materialize an agency independent of our intentions toward them" (57). Two years later, Diana Coole and Samantha Frost introduced their widely influential collection, New Materialisms: Ontology, Agency, and Politics, by announcing that it was time to "reopen the issue of matter and once again give material factors their due in shaping society and circumscribing human prospects" (3). A number of recent publications in rhetoric studies explain the variety of approaches one might take in this task of giving objects their due, and so I am not going to reproduce that effort here.[6] The salient point for us now is one that S. Scott Graham makes in his 2015 The Politics of Pain Medicine—namely that at the heart of the various manifestations that the ontological turn might take is a "diagnostic consensus" about the "two-world problem" that arises through the modernist bifurcation of subjects and objects (17). As Graham notes, identifying the separation of subjects and objects as problematic is not enough to make the ontological turn truly distinctive. Postmodern theory and its philosophical forbearers have long rejected the "litany of dualisms" that have characterized the Western intellectual tradition since Descartes, but they have not, Graham argues following Levi Bryant, been able to overcome the epistemic and hegemonic fallacies that stem from those dualisms (17–18). In brief, these fallacies are, one, that the absolute separation of subject and object "forces a constant reengagement" with questions of the subject's access to and representations of the object (the epistemic fallacy), and, two, that in a reversal of modernism's privileging of the object over the subject, postmodernism recasts the object "as an extension of the subject's perception," making it "an epiphenomenon of the subject" (the hegemonic fallacy) (19). In other words, then, what makes the ontological turn new is its rejection of not just the subject/object split but also the idea that, on account of this split, all we can ever hope for is what Kant set out for us over two hundred years ago with his Copernican Revolution: an understanding of the natural world that it based on how the mind (or culture) knows it.

What's interesting about this rejection of Kant's Copernican Revolution and the concomitant effort to begin giving the object its due is that both have an important historical precedent in our field. Scot Barnett makes this point in his 2016 *Rhetorical Realism: Rhetoric, Ethics, and the Ontology of Things*, a book that looks back to three periods in rhetorical history (antiquity, the early modern period, and the late twentieth century) to show that rhetoric has always engaged with the reality of objects, even in its most antirealist moments, for instance, the rhetoric-as-epistemic movement. But the precedent I have in mind isn't indicative of any particular period per se, and, more important, it deals directly with the subject of this book, a fact that I am inclined to see as more than just coincidence. I am talking, of course, about the work of Celeste Condit, particularly the 1999 essay, "The Materiality of Coding: Rhetoric, Genetics, and the Matter of Life," in which she argued for a "proto-theory of linguistic materialism" that, unlike its predecessor theories (e.g., historical materialism), could begin to account for the link between language and physical materiality. Offering her own version of the "diagnostic consensus" described by Graham, Condit argued that critiques of both the discourse of genetics (i.e., its use of coding, communication, and blueprint metaphors) and rhetoric as immaterial and disembodied stem from the same "long-standing (and by now well-analyzed, e.g., by Harding) Western dualism between the real and the ideal, appearance and reality, the

word and the thing" (327). But our response to this problem has not been sufficient, Condit wrote, insofar as it has "succeeded merely in reversing the hierarchy" such that the sign takes precedent over the referent, leaving us with a
critique of Western dualisms that is "still tarnished by the structuralist version
of idealism" and that can in no way specify "what kind of material being language
might have or what relationships might be among the sign, its physicality, and
the other biosocial forces in humanity's universe" (329).

Condit's approach to this problem was to suggest, following Burke's argument in "What Are the Signs of What," that language works by essentializing
matter/form relationships from the "linguistic, social, and physical planes" into
perceived objects (332–3). In this view, the agency of language is respected, as it
acknowledges that histories of linguistic use, for example, greatly affect our
understandings of and interactions with objects. But there is no sense in which
language creates objects *ex nihilo* since it must always "grapple with a social-
material universe that resists our rearrangement of it" (333). Thus, while we can
view rhetoric as constructive according to this theory, we are also left with "a
relatively solid universe" (333) where objects are "provisional but real" (334).
Condit illustrated this view through a number of examples from the natural
world, of which the most pertinent for our purposes is the gene (333). According
to her, the term *gene* identifies a discrete object for the purposes of scientific
communication, but no such object actually exists. Instead, what we call a gene
is a "set of overlapping relationships between materials and forms that serves
specific functions," most obviously that of coding for proteins (334). In her estimation, then, the gene "provides a paradigmatic example of the way in which
language constructs an objectified essence where none exists in nature—but
where that objectification is useful and is related to real material processes of
undeniable significance—and thus provides a terministic screen that both
enables and misleads" (334). In this sense, the term *gene* (and language in general) codes for meaning in much the same way the four nucleic acids of DNA do
so for proteins—that is by combining in nonarbitrary but also constricted ways
form/matter relationships that are useful, materially real, and yet nonessential
insofar as different combinations will produce different results (338).

Condit's early effort to find a way within rhetoric to begin giving objects their
due doesn't match up perfectly with more recent materialist work in our field,
especially if we agree that her argument stems more from a concern with the
materiality of language than with the materiality of things. But insofar as one of
her key claims is that no truly material theory of language can ignore physical

materiality, it does, I think, lead us to a similar conclusion about why critique
fails to produce the results we want it to—namely, because it doesn't just get the
subject wrong but also the object, reducing it to what society has made of it and
failing to see that even if it doesn't exist in any essential way, it is nonetheless real
(332). This view comes through in Condit's analysis of the discourses surrounding genetics, particularly in her claim that while the public forms of that discourse have been hampered by an "aporetic stasis" (that is, by a conflict between
genetic medicine's aim to control the human body and certain limits that make
such control impossible), the "critical discourse in response to that aporia has
been no wiser" (350). What Condit is talking about here are the ways in which
critics have responded to scientists' conflicted and often overblown claims about
the revolutionary potential of genetic medicine. Yes, those claims tend to "ignore
the significance and problems raised by the interfaces of the gene and by knowledge of the gene in our lives" but so do critiques of those claims, as they have
more often than not "simply sought to deny the criticality of the role of genes in
the body" (350–51). In other words, if science has erred by trying to march ahead
with no way of accounting for the social impacts and limitations of genetic
medicine, then its critics have erred in the opposite direction by focusing so
intently on social impacts that they can no longer recognize the distinction
between physical materiality, which does exist, and objective reality, which, as
they rightly argue, does not exist (332). The result on both sides, Condit argued,
is "an understanding of codes that is immaterial and arhetorical" (351).

Condit didn't elaborate this aspect of her argument (the problems with
critique) in "The Materiality of Coding"; nor did she apply it to the critiques of
choice that had made me rethink my initial response to those troublesome
aspects of the FORCE website. But still it served as an important impetus for
that rethinking, highlighting for me the problems that arise when we fail to
understand the objects that interest and trouble us as both provisional *and* real.
While critiques of choice provided compelling explanations of the social functions of genetic risk, it seemed to me that they did so at the expense of being
able to account for the realities of risk and the constraints imposed on BRCA+
women by those realities. And further it seemed that this inability made those
critiques unpersuasive. How would exposing BRCA risk as a set of heterosexist gender norms, for example, empower BRCA+ women to choose more
freely? It wouldn't, in my view, because that—heterosexist gender norms—was
not what BRCA risk was. Or at least that was not something BRCA risk could
be reduced to.

The challenge, then, became one of responding differently, of not accepting genetic medicine's promises of better health through personal choice but also not making the debunking of those promises the primary goal. As I have already indicated, Mol's delineation of care as an alternative to choice, one that "contains more suitable repertoires for handling life with a disease" (*The Logic of Care* 2), was my key resource for responding to this challenge. I recognized that handling life with a risk of disease was not the same thing as handling life with disease, yet it seemed to me that Mol's notion of care, with its emphasis on what patients do to live a good life when what they want (to not be patients) is out of reach, was precisely the right place to start thinking about the ideas and ideals from which an alternative rhetoric could be built. But it wasn't just Mol's notion of care that influenced my thinking. Also at work was the version articulated by Bruno Latour in his oft-cited 2004 essay, "Why Has Critique Run Out of Steam?" If objects of science and technology were not as susceptible to our social explanations as we once thought, then it was time to begin redirecting our critical capacities, Latour argued, time to retool by engaging those objects in such a way as to care for and protect them, not debunk them (232). The goal of criticism, in other words, was not to "pull the rug from beneath the feet of the naïve believers" but rather to assemble or compose, giving the "participants an arena in which to gather" and adding to the reality of the objects that mattered to them, not subtracting from it (246, 232). Although rhetoric had demonstrated well its ability to subtract reality from objects of science and technology, it seemed to me that its critical apparatus could be just as effective at adding it, provided that we did not then claim that reality was rhetorical. Thus, the rhetoric of care that I began to envision was one where the term *care* indicated not just an alternative choice but also an alternative to critique, to the idea that the best way to get close to BRCA risk was to debunk and demystify it.

Chapter Outline

I begin laying the groundwork for this rhetoric of care in chapter 1, "Following Mol's Lead: From Diabetes to BRCA Risk," where I review *The Logic of Care*, beginning with Mol's notion of care and the fact that it is not meant to evoke ideas of TLC but rather to call attention to how patients try to live a good life despite the fact that they are not free to choose what they want (5, 30). I then turn to how Mol understands the problem of choice in both its market and civic versions, what she aims to accomplish by offering a logic of care as an alternative to these versions of choice, and how she creates that logic through her fieldwork in a diabetes outpatient clinic in the Netherlands. My review of *The Logic of Care* is not comprehensive, but it is meant to be thorough enough for readers to understand how my efforts to create a rhetoric of care both build on and deviate from Mol's work. Those efforts, I should note, are the subject of chapter 4, and so while I do begin laying the groundwork for a rhetoric of care in this first chapter, I don't return to it again until after making some necessary deviations through constructivist and praxiographic understandings of genetic risk in chapters 2 and 3.

In addition to reviewing *The Logic of Care*, chapter 1 provides an introduction to BRCA risk, the other topic with which readers need some familiarity in order to follow my efforts to create a rhetoric of care. Introducing BRCA risk in this context means, first of all, recognizing how it differs from diabetes, the disease at the center of Mol's study. While I believe that rhetorics and logics of care are just as warranted in the case of genetic risk as they are in that of disease, I am also aware that the stakes of my endeavor are different from those of Mol's. I try to be upfront about these differences, acknowledging, for instance, that any attempt to craft a rhetoric of care for the at risk carries the potential of further muddying the line between health and illness that has drawn the attention of so many critics. I also try to provide readers with a basic explanation of the role of BRCA mutations in carcinogenesis. Though this explanation is, in fact, quite basic (owing to the fact that I am not a molecular biologist), I believe it is necessary because it provides important context for understanding the National Comprehensive Cancer Network (NCCN) guidelines for managing BRCA risk, which, in turn, are key to understanding the biosocial discourses surrounding BRCA risk. Finally, and in relation to the nondirective nature of these NCCN guidelines, I describe the rhetoric of choice that operates in those biosocial discourses, working under the assumption that if I am going to frame a rhetoric of care as an alternative to choice, then I should give readers a sense of what choice looks like and how it functions rhetorically.

Serving as the literature review and problem statement of this book, chapter 2, "From Ideology to Governmentality: A Constructivist View of Genetic Risk," reviews responses to this rhetoric of choice, focusing specifically on constructivist critiques of genetic medicine and genetic risk and arguing that they are organized, either explicitly or implicitly, around one of two key concepts:

ideology or governmentality. In the case of the former, critics typically claim that genetic science and medicine serve an ideological function by naturalizing dominant ideas about race, gender, and class and then seek to explain how various discourses mask that function. Insofar as the only thing to which these critiques grant any reality are the hidden ideological forces they seek to expose, I argue that they illustrate what Latour describes as the problem with the "fact position." This problem, in turn, means that even in critiques that take a very strong constructivist position, arguing that since everything is the product of discursive forces, there is no chance of seeing things as they "really are," an appearance/reality distinction emerges, placing the critic in the roles of decoder and debunker. I explain that in theory, analyses of genetic risk based on the concept of governmentality should avoid this problem (and the critical roles it creates). However, because most governmentality-based critiques of genetic risk tend to take strong constructivist positions on the nature of risk, questions about hidden purposes reemerge, placing objects like genetic risk in the fact position just as much as ideology critique. I demonstrate this pattern in chapter 2 by reviewing critiques that employ both concepts, ideology and governmentality. In the first half of the chapter, I focus on ideology, turning to a number of early critiques that warned of the oppressive, eugenic ideologies operating within genetic science and medicine. I then turn to the argument about hereditarian ideology and BRCA mutations that Kelly Happe makes in chapter 3 of her 2013 book, *The Material Gene: Gender, Race, and Heredity After the Human Genome Project*. I focus on Happe's argument here not only because it demonstrates how ingrained and repetitive the moves of ideology critique have become by 2013 but also what they yield in the particular context of genetic risk for breast and ovarian cancers. The second half of the chapter unfolds somewhat differently. Here I illustrate how the concept of governmentality has been used to understand genetic risk for breast and ovarian cancers by reviewing four studies, two of cancer diagnostic practices by Nina Hallowell and Press et al., and two of cancer prevention practices by Shona Crabb and Amanda LeCouteur and Tasha Dubriwny. However, I do more to contextualize these studies, beginning with a description of the concept of governmentality in the work of Foucault and other governmentality scholars and then moving to an explanation of where and how it has merged with constructivist views of risk to produce a kind of critique that still pivots around the appearance/reality distinction.

Chapter 3, "Making Risk Real: A Praxiographic Inquiry into Being BRCA+," marks the beginning of my response to these critiques and thus also to my effort to foster a rhetoric of care for the at risk. However, there isn't much talk of rhetoric in this chapter. As its title suggests, chapter 3 is a praxiographic study of BRCA risk, that is, a study of how the practices through which BRCA risk is enacted make it real. If we were to take up Latour's call to redirect our critical capacities, to treat the objects that interested us as matters of concern rather than matters of fact, then it seemed to me that we needed a way of understanding BRCA risk as something other than a social construction. It seemed to me, in other words, that if we always began with the idea that risks didn't exist in reality but instead were ways of crafting reality, that they were a category of the understanding, as Kant would have put it, then we would remain locked in the role of debunker, tasked automatically with the job of identifying the social forces at work behind the scenes of the appearance of reality. We needed, then, to begin with another idea about risk, one that would grant it some reality without reinscribing the culture/nature hierarchy, only this time with the second term on top. That I turned to praxiography for this idea speaks to what we might call the Mol-centric nature of this book. If *The Logic of Care* helped me figure out how I wanted to respond to the problem of choice in the discourses surrounding BRCA risk, then Mol's earlier book, *The Body Multiple: Ontology in Medical Practice*, was an essential resource for conceptualizing and crafting that response. *The Body Multiple*, as many readers will know, is a praxiographic study of atherosclerosis, a common artery disease that Mol "follows" through a hospital in the Netherlands in order to study how it is enacted in multiple practices and how, on account of those practices, it has many realities, not one. My praxiographic study is meant to suggest the same thing, namely that since BRCA risk can be enacted through different practices, it can (and does) have different realities, realities that are no less real for being situated, multiple, and contingent. But since my objective is somewhat different from Mol's (and since my praxiographic study is a single chapter in a book, not an entire book), I focus on one set of practices, high-risk breast cancer screening, demonstrating how it "does" or enacts BRCA risk and the at-risk body and offering this demonstration as an example of how we can understand the reality of this messy medical object. My specific argument here, which is based on several types of biosocial discourse, including interviews with BRCA+ women and posts from the FORCE message boards, as well as medical texts such as research articles and patient guides, is that this set of practices does BRCA risk in such a way that risk and disease overlap, particularly through the problem of false positive test results on breast MRIs, a test that became part of the NCCN high-risk screening guidelines in 2009. I explain this problem in considerable detail in the second half of the chapter, ultimately arguing that it is precisely the kind of constraint in medicine that necessitates a rhetoric of care.

Chapter 4, "Toward a Rhetoric of Care for the At Risk," finally brings us to this rhetoric of care, though not without a somewhat lengthy preamble about the theoretical framework on which it is based. Indeed, almost the first third of the chapter serves as an explanation of what it means theoretically (and, to a lesser extent, historically) to argue for a move from hermeneutics to invention within RSTM scholarship, acknowledging, among other things, that such a move is complicated by the fact that the revitalization of invention in the mid-twentieth century paved the way for the use of rhetoric as a global hermeneutic. If rhetoric didn't just dress arguments but also invented them, the reasoning went, then arguments in any field could be understood in rhetorical terms. Recognizing that this kind of reverse engineering is always possible, I trace efforts within the recent history of rhetoric to "orient" (Muckelbauer, *The Future of Invention*) toward invention, focusing specifically on Richard McKeon's concept of an architectonic productive art, Janet Atwill's interpretation of the ancient Greek concept of *logon techne*, and John Muckelbauer's related notions of "productive reading" and "affirmative repetition." While these concepts are far from synonymous, I explain how elements of each can promote a form of inquiry where the goal is to invent, to read the rhetorics of choice that surround BRCA risk as a resource for creating a rhetoric of care. Looking back to *The Logic of Care*, I argue that while Mol positions her work in that book at the intersection of philosophy and the social sciences, it can also be understood as an act of rhetorical invention in this sense. I then turn to the four topics that compose this rhetoric of care, explaining how I see them functioning in rhetorics of choice and how I think they can be used to foster a rhetoric of care. Accompanying these explanations are a few caveats, the most important of which is the fact that I don't believe I (or anyone else) can simply create a rhetoric of care. A real rhetoric of care can only emerge over time, just as rhetorics of choice have done over decades of debate about genetic science and medicine. The goal of the four topics I offer, then, is to encourage that emergence by providing us with a new set of conceptual starting points.

Finally, the conclusion, "Invention in RSTM: Another Moderate Response to the Two-World Problem," considers the implications of the arguments made in *Being at Genetic Risk,* focusing specifically on the theoretical framework laid out in chapter 4 and drawing on Graham's argument about the relationship between rhetorical and new materialist theory to show how that framework can provide the basis of what he describes as a more "moderate" but also "more fully interventional" form of "rhetorical-ontological inquiry."

1

Following Mol's Lead | From Diabetes to BRCA Risk

In 1974, when I was about one year old, my mother found a lump in her breast. I know very few details about this event, only that because of her age (thirty-two) and lack of family history, doctors thought the lump was benign but went ahead and ordered an excisional biopsy, a procedure that at that time was done under general anesthesia. Histological testing performed while she was asleep revealed that the lump was malignant. As a result, a mastectomy was performed, and my mother woke from anesthesia to find out not only that she had breast cancer but also that her left breast had been removed. She was not offered and did not receive any adjuvant therapy and lived for more than a decade without a recurrence. When the cancer did return in 1986, she underwent radiation and chemotherapy for three years and then died in 1989.

Thirty-nine years later, in the spring of 2015, when I was forty years old and well into research for this book, a regular screening mammogram led to a diagnosis of ductal carcinoma in situ, or DCIS. As far as breast cancer diagnoses go, DCIS is a good one because the cancerous breast cells are confined to the milk ducts and have not yet developed the ability to invade surrounding tissue. At my first consultation with my breast surgeon, I was given two surgical options, lumpectomy or mastectomy. My surgeon explained the pros and cons of both procedures in great and well-rehearsed detail, working hard to provide unbiased accounts, even though I could tell that she had a clear preference about which option I should choose. Thankfully, at this stage of the treatment process, I, too, had a clear preference about which option I should choose. When I announced my decision, it was obvious to me that she thought I was making the right choice, yet she wouldn't come out and say that. Even if we were on the same page—and we were—she was to remain an unbiased provider of information, a facilitator of my right to choose freely.

Even without my surgeon's explicit affirmation, I proceeded through this part of treatment without much doubt or second-guessing. That was not to be

the case later on. Some issues with my surgery (it had gone well but not perfectly) had unexpectedly raised the possibility of adjuvant therapy, namely,
undergoing twenty-five whole-breast radiation treatments, taking the antiestro-
gen medication tamoxifen for at least five years, or doing both. These treatments
are not as toxic as chemotherapy, but they are no walk in the park, either. Radiation can damage your heart (and I would have needed it on my left breast), and
tamoxifen comes with a long and nasty list of possible side effects. If at the earlier stage of this decision-making process I had felt a good deal of clarity, then at
this stage I felt none. I did not know what to do. I did not know which—if
any—adjuvant therapy to choose. The only thing that was clear was that the
decision was *entirely* up to me. If I wanted the extra risk reduction provided by
radiation and/or tamoxifen, then it was available to me. All I had to do was ask,
to "pull the trigger" as one radiation oncologist so unpalatably put it. But, on the
other hand, if I declined these treatments because of the potential for negative
side effects, then that was perfectly fine, too. Current evidence-based medicine
supported this choice, and none of my doctors would have questioned it.

This offer of adjuvant cancer therapy created a very difficult decision-making
situation for me. The stakes in my decision were high, yet there was no right or
wrong choice. Figuring out what to do was essentially a matter of figuring out
what I wanted. But who really *wants* radiation or tamoxifen? Want, I came to
realize, was not a good criterion for making choices about cancer treatment. *But
at least I had choices, right?* In 1974, my mother had none. She went to sleep
thinking that the lump in her breast was benign and woke up with a mastectomy. She had no say about who performed her surgery or about what kind of
surgery it was. Compared to her ordeal, my experience of breast cancer and
breast cancer treatment is a shining example of the hard-won achievements of
the women's health movement. For my mother, that movement began just a
couple of years too late. She and Rose Kushner were diagnosed with breast
cancer the same year, and it was in large part because of Kushner's subsequent
work as a breast cancer activist that surgeons stopped conducting biopsies and
mastectomies as one-step surgical procedures. Kushner was also part of the
effort to establish simple mastectomies and lumpectomies as acceptable breast
cancer surgeries, thus helping to spare many women the disfigurement and dis-
ability of radical mastectomy (Lerner 178). There is no doubt that I am a benefi-
ciary of these and many other efforts to give breast cancer patients more control
over their health care. My situation—being able to choose between not just
lumpectomy and mastectomy but also between having adjuvant therapy and

not having it—would have been inconceivable in 1974. Of course my situation was better than my mother's for other reasons, too, namely improved biopsy and imaging techniques, better understanding of breast cancer, and, most important, a better diagnosis. But still, I was lucky to have choices, and so no matter how troubling my decision-making dilemma was, I would take that over the paternalism of 1970s medicine any day.

Obviously this preference does not make me unique. Most people prefer having choice to not having it, especially when it comes to their health. But what happens when choice is contrasted not to lack of choice but to *care*? As patients, what is more important to us—making free choices or receiving and participating in good care? This is the central question Annemarie Mol asks in *The Logic of Care: Health and the Problem of Patient Choice*. There she argues that while the critiques of medical power that began in the 1960s and 1970s were a necessary response to the hubris and paternalism of the medical establishment, they were also too narrowly focused on the tasks of unmasking and undermining (90). After exposing the problems of unquestioned medical authority, they offered nothing new to take its place, and the result was a hole in how we think about health care and what makes it good (90). To our detriment, the people who eventually filled that hole were the rationalists, and the thing they filled it with was the ideal of autonomous choice, an ideal that tells us health care is good when it is freely chosen by patients who have the monetary resources and/or knowledge necessary for informed decision making. To be clear, Mol does not believe that it is bad for patients to have choices. She is not after a return to the paternalism of the 1970s. But she does believe that as an organizing logic, choice does not capture what actually goes on in the interactions between patients and health-care professionals. At their best, those interactions are guided by a different logic, a logic of care that, though quite distinct from the logic of choice, is hard to recognize because we lack a language for describing it. Mol's goal in *The Logic of Care*, then, is to craft such a language. In other words, she wants to give us a way of thinking and talking about what patients actually *do* in order to live a good life when what they really want (to not be sick) is out of reach.

As I explained in the introduction, my goal in this book is to follow in Mol's lead, adopting and adapting her work in order to create a rhetoric of care for those at genetic risk of breast and ovarian cancers due to a BRCA mutation. The purpose of this chapter is to provide some of the background necessary for that task. Thus, in the first part of the chapter, I review *The Logic of Care*, explaining what Mol means by the term *care*, how she uses fieldwork in a diabetes outpatient clinic to articulate a logic of care, and some of the ways in which she positions this logic as an alternative to the two versions of choice that dominate health care in the West, the market version and the civic version. Although *The Logic of Care* is a slender volume, just 129 pages in all, it is not an easy book to summarize. Part of Mol's argument in *The Logic of Care* is that good care cannot be generalized but rather is specific to particular diseases, institutions, and locations. Thus, her ideas about the logic of care, which are primarily based on interviews and observations at a diabetes outpatient clinic in the Netherlands, are presented more by way of example than exposition. I include a number of those examples here, but my summaries of them can only gesture toward the more vivid pictures painted in Mol's text. In the second half of the chapter, I turn from *The Logic of Care* to the actual object of investigation in this book, BRCA risk, briefly explaining how researchers understand the role that these two genes play in carcinogenesis, the estimated lifetime risk of developing cancer that BRCA1 and 2 mutations confer, and the current surveillance and risk-reduction guidelines given to BRCA+ women. The aim in this part of the chapter is twofold: again, I want to give readers the information that they need to follow arguments later in the book, but I also want to make clear some of the ways in which this object of investigation differs from the one at the center of Mol's study (diabetes). BRCA risk is not a disease but rather a genetic predisposition for disease. It is hard to overestimate the significance of this difference for a project like this. Among other things, it means that that choice is essential in this health-care context. Importantly, that is not to say that choice is real (i.e., not an illusion) or even that it is good (though it is hard to make the case that choice is bad). Rather, to say that choice is essential in the context of genetic risk is to say that because it functions as the most visible marker between eugenics and the new genetics, it is fundamental to how health care is conceived by and delivered to people with BRCA mutations.[1] Thus, at the end of this chapter, I briefly describe the rhetoric of choice that operates within the biosocial discourses surrounding BRCA risk, showing how it corresponds in some key ways to Mol's civic version of the logic of choice.

From Choice to Care

I want to begin this review of Mol's work with the term at the center of it—*care*. As Mol repeatedly notes, *care* is a difficult term to pin down, particularly when it is preceded by the adjective *good*. Indeed, this difficulty is one way of under-standing the exigence of her book: the logic of choice so thoroughly dominates health care in the West that we don't have an adequate language for talking about what counts as good care. But what, in general terms, does *care* mean for Mol? Outside the context of a specific disease, it is easier to begin answering this question by saying what *care* does not mean for Mol. She does not use the term, for instance, to refer to what we might think of as "tender loving care." Nor does she use it to conjure up images from a pre-technological past; *care* is not, as she puts it, "a pre-modern remainder in a modern world" (5). Moreover, *care* is not romantic or something we can easily romanticize; it is not always attractive or appreciated; and it is certainly not opposed to those developments we have come to understand under the umbrella term "medicalization." Rather *care*, in a general sense, is best understood very simply as what patients do to make daily life with a medical condition more bearable (1). This is why the term is so often followed by "practices" in *The Logic of Care*; Mol wants us to focus on what it is that patients do in order to live a good life when what they really want—perfect health—is not possible. Understood in these terms, it is tempting to contrast *care* with *cure*, thinking that while care practices make life better on a daily basis, cures intervene and heal. Mol rejects this distinction, however, arguing that in the twenty-first century, when so many of the health problems that send people to their doctors are chronic conditions, care and cure overlap. Much of what goes under the name "cure" doesn't completely heal but instead makes day-to-day life better (10).

In light of this understanding of care, it is easy to see why Mol chose diabetes as her test case for articulating a logic of care. Insofar as diabetes patients depend on industrially made injectable insulin to survive, their lives are intimately tied up with modern medical technology. Thus, it is hard to think of diabetes care as a "pre-modern 'care remnant' in an otherwise modern world" or to simply "dis-card" medicalization as an unwarranted encroachment of medicine into all fac-ets of life (10). Moreover, diabetes is a chronic disease; patients cannot be cured, but if they regularly and actively participate in care practices, then their chances of living a good life are high. In this context, then, it would be fair to say that there aren't many choices to be made, but there is a lot of caring to be done; and much of that caring is self-caring. Diabetes patients must regularly test their blood sugar levels, inject their own insulin, monitor their nutrition, and cali-brate their exercise (7). And what's more, Mol points out, is that a great deal of this caring—both that done by physicians and that done by patients—takes place through medical practices that are well understood and "overtly attended to," which means that they are accessible and can be studied without too much difficulty (11).

As I noted earlier, Mol's method for studying these practices was largely ethnographic. Working as a participant-observer in the diabetes outpatient clinic of a university hospital in a medium-sized Dutch town, she was able to observe consultations between health-care professionals and their patients, gain access to a variety of diabetes-related texts, and conduct interviews with a wide range of participants (9). Through all of these methods of data collection, Mol's objective was not to assess participants' opinions about life with diabetes but instead to learn about the events and activities they participated in so that she could identify the logics underlying them (9). She then explains that logic, the logic of care, primarily by way of comparison, demonstrating how it and the two versions of choice that dominate health care in the West—the market version and the civic version—differ across a wide range of issues related to diabetes treatment. In the first part of this demonstration, she treats each version of choice separately, explaining its key features and then using those features as points of contrast for the logic of care. She then turns to features shared by the two versions of choice, again using them as a foil for fleshing out the logic of care. While I cannot include all of Mol's argument in this review, I do want to provide enough explanation that readers have a good sense of how she understands these two logics. To that end, I have focused my review on six of the issues Mol discusses, two that relate to the market version of choice, two that relate to the civic version, and two that relate to both versions.

The Market Version of Choice

Generally speaking, the market version of choice understands patients as customers who buy their care in exchange for money and are entitled to a certain value for their expenditure (14). In addition, and since this version is based on the idea of a market, it is the patient who determines demand, not the doctor. Thus, there is a sense in which the patient, as a customer, is always right. Or, to borrow Burger King's longtime advertising slogan, we might say that according to the market version of choice, you can "have it your way" in the clinic as long as you know what you want and can pay for it. Put in these terms, it is easy to see why Mol believes that the market version of choice is a poor fit for health care. Patients are not always right; they often do not know what they want; and want is not necessarily a good criterion for making decisions about health. Moreover, Mol argues that embedded in this logic is a particularly problematic notion of what it is that health care offers. In the market version of choice, patients are customers who choose, and so it stands to reason they must have something to choose; thus, health care is thought to provide a product, something that has a beginning and an end and can be differentiated from other products (20). Mol concedes that a lot might be included in this product, for instance services, training for using the product, and even "kindness and attention," but still what is "on offer" has to be specified so that the customer can choose it or not choose it (18).

In the consultation room, however, Mol observes something different. The aim of care in the case of diabetes is to help people regulate their blood sugar, a function their bodies cannot properly carry out any longer. At first, this task requires considerable teaching and assistance, as nurses inject insulin for patients and technicians measure their blood sugar levels. But eventually patients or machines (e.g., an insulin pump) take over the work, and the nature of the task, as well as the kind of care it involves, shifts, hopefully in such a way that patients are doing more of it (and so therefore coming to the hospital less) and using (or buying) less "product" (18–19). In other words, the hope is that patients will learn how to measure blood sugar levels so well that they can fine-tune the dose of insulin, getting it as low as possible (19). But things don't always work that way; bodies are unpredictable and even good care can fail to produce good results. "It follows from this unpredictability," Mol writes, "that good care is not a well-delineated product, but an open-ended process" (20). Good care, she elaborates, does not have clear boundaries and does not even determine who does which task since various people, instruments, and machines must work together over time toward a result. Contrary to what the logic of choice tells us, care is "not a transaction in which something is exchanged (a product against a price), but an interaction, an ongoing process that doesn't end until the patient dies" (20).

If, in the logic of care, health care is an open-ended process that ends only when life does, then it stands to reason that perfect health is not what it aims for or what it teaches patients to aim for. That sounds counterintuitive insofar as the aim of all health care should be to diminish illness and increase health. To an extent, Mol agrees that this is what health care should aim for, but she is troubled by the degree to which the market version of choice plays on patient desire for health, using only positive terms and often suggesting that if only the right products are purchased, then health can be brought within reach (26). This way of thinking makes sense within a logic of choice, where more desire leads to more purchases and more purchases lead to more health. But in real life, and particularly in the case of a chronic illness like diabetes, health care doesn't work this way. No matter how much care diabetes patients purchase, Mol writes, they will never be free of disease and all the complications and interferences it entails. So if the logic of care does not teach patients to hope for health then what does it teach them? What does it tell them to aim for? Rather simply, it suggests that the goal for patients is to learn to live with disease, accepting that they are patients and they have a disease they did not choose to have (28). Learning to live with disease doesn't mean patients should be reduced to their disease or that they should be encouraged to give up, Mol points out (26). But it does mean that they should be realistic, "striving for improvement while respecting the erratic nature of disease" (27).

To illustrate the difference between hoping for health and living with disease, Mol recounts a consultation between a diabetes nurse and a patient, Mrs. Jansen, who had just been diagnosed and was learning how to measure her blood sugar levels. Mol observed the nurse as she instructed Mrs. Jansen to always prick her finger on the side, never on the fingertip. In learning how to measure her blood sugar levels, Mrs. Jansen was learning a strategy for preventing or delaying the complications of diabetes, which can include blindness. But, as Mol explains, the nurse taught Mrs. Jansen to prick the sides of her finger rather than the tops so that if she does go blind, she can use the tops to feel the world around her. "Thus at the very moment when one learns how to prick," Mol writes, "there is hope of health as well as acceptance of disease. You learn how to prick so that you may stay healthy for as long as possible. But you respect the fact that the reality of disease is erratic by practically anticipating the complications, blindness included, that may occur even so" (27).

The Civic Version of Choice

The civic version of choice is similar to the market version to the extent that both prioritize the act of choosing over all others. Beyond this similarity, though, Mol sees them as quite different. Within the civic version of choice, patients are citizens rather than customers, and that means that choice is understood primarily in the language of rights and responsibilities, not products and preferences. This language is visibly displayed in many exam rooms in the West in the form of posters that itemize patients' rights, telling them, for instance, that they are entitled to as much information about a particular treatment or procedure as they need and demanding in return (even if only implicitly) that they share all relevant information about their condition (29). As Mol explains, the goal of this language and the logic it embodies is to balance the scales between patients and professionals, that is, to put an end to the era of doctors having near complete power and authority over their patients. By becoming citizens endowed with rights and responsibilities, patients were to be emancipated, made the equals of the physicians whose care they sought (30).

On the face of it, this shift to the language of citizenship seems like a step in the right direction. After all, citizens are not lorded over by "patriarchal rulers" but instead operate according to a contract that "stipulates that they are masters of their own lives" (30). But even if this language and the logic it embodies mark an improvement over the past, Mol does not consider them to be a good fit for health care. To be a citizen, she argues, is to be unfettered by one's body or to have a body that does not interfere with one's plans or one's ability to make rational choices. In fact, it is precisely because citizens' bodies are "silent" that they can make their own choices (31). Moreover, the notion of emancipation that is built into the idea of citizenship is, in Mol's estimation, a very limited ideal in the context of health care, one that misunderstands the relationships between patients and physicians and obscures the fact that often patients cannot be liberated from what oppresses them the most—disease. Mol elaborates:

> If you have a potentially lethal disease and there is a drug like insulin that is likely to allow you to live for quite a while longer, what do you do? When they talk about this, most patients say: "I have no choice." But this lack of choice does not call for emancipation. That they feel no freedom is not because they have been submitted to the force of an authority. Something else is going on. Once dead, you have no choices left at all. (40)

After introducing the civic version of choice broadly, in terms of this limited ideal of emancipation, Mol turns to predominant notions of citizenship in political theory, aiming not to explain them in any kind of technical detail but rather to use them as focal points for highlighting specific differences between the logic of care and the civic version of choice. The first comparison she develops, for instance, focuses on the common notion of a citizen as someone who is civilized, that is, someone who displays bourgeois values insofar as he or she is capable of taming the passions and keeping "bodily behavior" under control for the sake of "self-rule" and clear, rational thinking (34). Even without much explanation, we can imagine how life with a disease like diabetes could provide a strong counterargument about the value of this notion of citizenship in health-care contexts. Diabetes affects not just a patient's physical well-being but also his or her cognitive abilities. When its blood sugar levels are too high or too low, a diabetic body gets in the way of "self-rule" and clear, rational thinking. The patients Mol observed often reported to their physicians that they worried about getting "hypos" (episodes of hypoglycemia) in public for this very reason, namely that they might call attention to themselves by saying something strange or being too aggressive. Yet they also reported being reluctant to eat in such situations for fear that it, too, would draw unwanted attention to their bodies (35). The bottom line, in Mol's view, is that controlling bodily behavior is not easy for a diabetic (or for anyone who is sick) and therefore should not be the basis on which a patient is taken seriously or not.

Rather than aiming to tame or control our bodies, then, a logic of care seeks to nourish them. In the broadest sense, to nourish means to acknowledge, as doctors do in the consulting room, that the body is not just what a patient speaks about but also the basis from which he or she speaks (35). In addition, though, Mol writes that nourishing the body also means accepting that passions and bodily desire for pleasure are a normal and important part of life, even life with disease. Of course diabetes is a disease that demands moderation when it comes to pleasures like alcohol and sweets, but Mol points out this demand for moderation has nothing to do with asceticism. Diabetics shouldn't watch their consumption of alcohol and sugar because pleasure is bad but instead because overconsumption now could lead to complications that interfere with other pleasures in the future (36). Within a logic of care, professionals recognize that pleasure is not in and of itself bad, and they don't castigate those patients who have not followed the dietary rules as closely as they should have. Instead, for those patients they try to identify the obstacles to good care while teaching them that even if that care meddles with and tries to normalize their bodies, it does not despise or repress them (37).

Another notion of citizenship to which Mol contrasts the logic of care is the enlightened citizen. Like civilized citizens, enlightened citizens are not bothered by their bodies, but instead of trying to control them, they aim to escape them by gaining the "reflective distance" necessary for making critical, autonomous judgments (37). The goal here, in other words, is to be a free spirit, that is, someone who understands the causal links through which a body "hangs together" and who can apply that understanding without getting bogged down in "disturbing physicalities." As Mol points out, though, "disturbing physicalities" tend to draw patients into their bodies, and often those physicalities don't conform to causal explanations about the ways in which bodies work (37). Or even if they do, they might not be that helpful. Increasing blood sugar, for instance, causes a body to produce insulin, which in turn causes the cells to absorb sugar. This causal chain makes sense, but Mol argues that it doesn't capture what goes on in the consulting room, where the goal is not first and foremost to understand why something is happening but rather to figure out how best to intervene. In the consulting room, in other words, technical interventions matter more than natural laws (38). So while the logic of choice might seek to mobilize knowledge from the natural sciences in the clinic, the logic of care puts that knowledge in the service of the practical task of determining what should be done, acknowledging that "bodies are not trapped in causal chains" but instead "are embedded in treatment practices" (38).

Mol illustrates this difference between the two logics with a story about a patient, Mrs. Alzari, who drinks an excessive four liters of water a day. During Mrs. Alzari's consultation, Mol observed that the doctor's interest in her excessive thirst wasn't related to what it revealed about the nature of her disease, that is, what was happening under her skin to cause excessive thirst; rather, she was interested in the treatment practices it pointed to and, in particular, what those practices would demand of Mrs. Alzari. Yes, the doctor would be the one to order the tests necessary for figuring out how to deal with Mrs. Alzari's excessive thirst, but Mrs. Alzari herself would have to actively participate in that process, passing urine, giving blood, and eventually injecting her own insulin and developing the ability to "intro-sense," that is to feel a "hypo" coming on before it becomes a problem (39). This kind of participation is the opposite of being a free spirit; it is embodied and active, demanding a "physical competence" from patients who don't transcend their bodies but instead inhabit them (39).

Choice Versus Care More Broadly

These, then, are the two versions of choice that dominate health care in the West and some of the issues that differentiate them from the logic of care. The market version of choice treats health care as a product and teaches patients to hope for health, while the logic of care treats health care as a process and teaches patients how to live with disease. The civic version of choice promotes various notions of citizenship, for instance, the notion of the civilized citizen who tames her body and that of the enlightened citizen who understands how it works, while the logic of care promotes a vision of patients who live in their bodies and accept their limitations and failings, even as they strive for good health. Even though these two versions of choice play out very differently in actual health-care situations, they are linked by a number of similarities, which Mol examines in two chapters of *The Logic of Care*, again working by way of contrast to flesh out the logic of care that she seeks to promote. In a chapter titled "Managing and Doctoring," for instance, she argues that both versions of choice treat scientific knowledge as a collection of "informative facts" that doctors disseminate to patients when a decision needs to be made. In this way of thinking, doctors are responsible for facts, which come first, and patients are responsible for adding in the values, which come second. Once facts and values have been combined, the patient makes a choice (since it is his or her life that will be affected) and the doctor implements it through various medical technologies. Actually dispensing and receiving health care is, of course, a much messier process, one where facts and values are intertwined and technologies complicate treatment plans as much as they simply implement them. Thus, Mol contrasts the notion of "informative facts" to that of "target values," arguing that in the logic of care what counts as a medical or scientific fact cannot be determined outside of the context of care practices. Even in the case of something as straightforward as blood sugar levels, facts do not precede decisions about how to intervene. This is true, Mol observes, in both the consulting room and in the medical literature, where understandings of acceptable blood sugar levels fluctuate according to the specific situation (or audience) at hand (45). Target values, then, are what doctors aim for, and they do this *during* the treatment process, not before it. In other words, determining a target value doesn't allow doctors to act but instead is part of what they do when they act (46). Moreover, target values do not emerge, as informative facts do, solely from knowledge about diseases and bodies, but instead they deal with patients' lives, extending beyond care practices to those practices that affect work, family, school, friends, and so on (46). What follows from this broader view, Mol argues, "is that for the logic of care, gathering knowledge is not a matter of providing better maps *of* reality, but of crafting more bearable ways of living *with* or *in* reality" (46; emphasis added).

The final point of difference between these two logics that I will review here has to do with fluidity, specifically where each logic locates fluidity in the health-care process. In the logic of choice, fluidity is located primarily in the moment of choosing, when facts are laid out and possible courses of action are considered (50). Such an understanding of fluidity suggests that the task at hand is one of calculating: in order to make a choice, patients, with the aid of their physicians, must perform a kind of cost-benefit analysis that takes into account their preferences and their predictions about what treatments will work. In contrast, the logic of care locates fluidity throughout the treatment process, not in the moment of choice. Patients tend to want a lot, Mol writes, but facts, habits, other people, technologies, and material conditions often refuse to bend to their will (53). Thus, there are limits to what can be changed or achieved, and these limits are not always obvious or predictable at the beginning, when patients are contemplating what they want (53). In the logic of care, then, the task at hand is not one of calculating but instead one of attuning, that is, of experimenting carefully throughout the treatment process in order to achieve the best outcome within a specific set of constraints.

To illustrate the difference between calculating and attuning, Mol describes a patient, Mr. Zoomer, who fails to regularly record his blood sugar levels, despite knowing that this practice can prevent complications like blindness. In the logic of choice, his failure would be seen as the outcome of a cost-benefit analysis that ended with his decision not to record levels (52–53). But the interaction that Mol observed between Mr. Zoomer and his caregivers pointed to something else. Trying to "disentangle the practicalities" of the patient's daily life, the doctor discovered that Mr. Zoomer's construction job provides few opportunities for recording blood sugar levels. A nurse then recommended that he measure once a day for five days rather than five times once a day. In the logic of care, then, the patient's failure (which indicates little about what he wants or if he is free to choose) leads to an effort to attune, that is, to make adjustments that will make daily life with diabetes more bearable (53).

It would be fair to say that making daily life more bearable is the goal of the logic of care in general, not just this aspect of it that Mol identifies as "attuning." However, by way of concluding this review, I should point out that when Mol identifies practices that have the potential to achieve this goal, she is not implicitly endorsing the quality of care that most people receive. In other words, she is not suggesting that, as it stands, most people receive good care. Nor is she claiming that the logic of care is in every way and in every instance superior to the logic of choice (83). In her view, its strengths stem primarily from its emphasis on patients as people who act rather than people who choose. Being able to choose was supposed to emancipate patients, but Mol argues that its real accomplishment has been to obscure the fact that patients act even though they are not free to choose (82). What her logic of care aims to do, then, is to give us a way of talking about this kind of constrained acting so that we can begin to improve health care in its own terms, not those of the market or of political theory (84). Of course Mol admits that no single logic of care can do this for every health care context, and so her parting challenge to readers in *The Logic of Care* is to extend her work, not "absorb[ing] it passively, but us[ing] it actively" to figure out what changes and what stays the same when we move into new contexts (90).

Care in the Context of BRCA Risk

This, then, is the task that I have set out for myself—to take Mol's work into a new context and use it as a model for creating not another logic of care but instead a rhetoric of care. Later in the book, I will explain how I understand this difference between Mol's preferred term, logic, and mine, rhetoric. For now, though, I want to focus on another key difference, namely the fact that the context I want to move into (that of BRCA risk) is not the context of a disease but rather that of a genetic predisposition to disease. Had I tried, I probably could not have chosen a context that seems less similar to the one at the center of Mol's study. As I explained earlier, she chose diabetes because it is a chronic disease characterized by a set of "overtly attended to" care practices that can be easily studied. Moreover, within diabetes care, there aren't many "bifurcation points," that is, situations that ask patients to make irreversible choices between irreconcilable options. This is what I meant earlier when I said that for diabetes patients, there aren't that many choices to be made, but there is a lot of caring to be done. BRCA risk is, in many ways, a very different story. First of all, it is not a disease. Many women with diagnosed BRCA mutations will take no risk-reducing action and live long, full, cancer-free lives.[2] Second, not only are the care practices associated with BRCA risk not "overtly attended to" in the same way that they are in diabetes care, but they are also very decentralized, spread over so many different types of health-care professionals that studying them in one location would be next to impossible. And third, while there is quite a lot of caring to be done in the case of BRCA risk (a fact that surprises some people), there are also unavoidable, sometimes irreversible choices that must be made;

and, to return to a point I made at the outset of this chapter, it is precisely because BRCA risk is not a disease that these choices—or, rather, *the fact that there are choices*—must remain front and center in this health-care context. Thus, even if my goal is to articulate a rhetoric of care for those at genetic risk of breast and ovarian cancers, I have to acknowledge that this is a health-care context that cannot function without a logic—*and a rhetoric*—of choice. Later in this chapter, I do this by describing the rhetoric of choice that operates in the biosocial discourses surrounding BRCA risk, a rhetoric that, as we will see, corresponds quite closely with the civic version of the logic of choice as outlined by Mol. First, though, I provide readers with some context for understanding this rhetoric by briefly explaining how researchers understand the role that BRCA mutations play in carcinogenesis, the kind of risk those mutations confer, and the current surveillance and risk-reduction guidelines given to BRCA+ women for managing or mitigating that risk.

BRCA Risk: An Introduction

Compared to other genes related to adult-onset disease, BRCA1 and 2 hardly need introducing. Books like *Breakthrough: The Race to Find the Breast Cancer Gene*; *The Breast Cancer Wars*; *What We Have*; *Pandora's DNA*; *Blood Matters*; *Leaving Long Island*; and *Pretty Is What Changes*—just to name a few—have documented and publicized the story of these two genes as it has played out in the labs of geneticists, the examination rooms of oncologists, gynecologists, and plastic surgeons, and the homes of those who have either inherited a BRCA mutation or been born into a family where one exists. In 2009, the story of BRCA1 and 2 began playing out in the courtroom, as Myriad Genetics tried but failed to defend its patent on the two genes, and in 2013, the same year the Supreme Court delivered its verdict against Myriad, Angelina Jolie published her first *New York Times* op-ed about being BRCA+ and her decision to have a risk-reducing bilateral mastectomy. She followed up in 2015 with another *New York Times* op-ed, this time detailing an ovarian cancer scare and her subsequent decision to have risk-reducing bilateral salpingo-oophorectomy. BRCA1 and 2 have been the subject of at least two films, Joanna Rudnick's 2008 documentary, *In the Family*, and the 2013 motion picture *Decoding Annie Parker*, which starred Helen Hunt as famed geneticist and BRCA2 discoverer, Mary-Claire King. Beyond what has been published or produced about the BRCA genes in the mainstream media, there is an incredibly robust biosocial community surrounding BRCA risk, one that encourages those affected by BRCA mutations to share their experiences through blogs, message boards, and other online mediums, as well as through in-person events like confer- ences and support groups. As I explained in the introduction, this community is led by FORCE, but other online organizations, for instance, Be Bright Pink and BRCA Umbrella, are a part of it, providing even more venues for BRCA+ women to seek and offer advice, to gain information, and to advocate for policies and research that affect them. With so many resources available, it can seem as though there is almost no aspect of the "BRCA experience" that one cannot find documented somewhere in some published form, be it online or in print.

The amount of attention given to the "BRCA experience" is not surprising in light of the culture that surrounds breast cancer in the West. There's no need for me to explain the details of that culture here; this task has been taken on by many before me in books like Barron Lerner's *The Breast Cancer Wars*; Audre Lorde's *The Cancer Journals*; Robert Aronowitz's *Unnatural History*; Maren Klawiter's *The Biopolitics of Breast Cancer*; and Gayle Sulik's *Pink Ribbon Blues*. The salient point here, and it is one that all of these books make in some fashion or another, is that at least since the 1970s, messages to prevent breast cancer through smart lifestyle choices or to catch it early through vigilant surveillance have been promulgated more persistently and more loudly than any other, creat- ing a situation in which individual women—not the companies that pollute, the manufacturers that make carcinogenic products, or the politicians who fail to improve people's economic and environmental conditions—are responsible for protecting themselves from this disease. Within a situation like this, the discov- ery of two genes linked to the development of breast cancer could not fail to garner a tremendous amount of attention. The idea of a genetic cause for breast cancer fit perfectly into the individual prevention and surveillance paradigm established by mainstream breast cancer culture, and so even if researchers repeatedly explained that only about 5 to 10 percent of breast cancers were thought to be related to genetic mutations, BRCA1 and 2 moved quickly into the national spotlight, as patients, advocates, and physicians sought to deter- mine and promote the steps that BRCA mutation carriers could take to be "proactive" with their health and prevent cancer rather than waiting for it to "strike." Indeed, these steps—primarily prophylactic bilateral mastectomy (PBM) and prophylactic bilateral salpingo-oophorectomy (PBSO)—have received significant media attention, as various groups of stakeholders have weighed in on the medical, psychosocial, ethical, and political issues that make the decision to have risk-reducing surgery such a fraught one.[3] What has received considerably less attention are the biological mechanisms by which researchers believe mutations in these genes contribute to carcinogenesis, as well as the tumor characteristics associated with BRCA-related breast and ovarian cancers. I provide a brief (and, to be clear, a lay) explanation of those mechanisms and characteristics here because I believe they are important context for understanding the National Comprehensive Cancer Network (NCCN) risk management guidelines for BRCA+ women. These guidelines, in turn, are important context for understanding the rhetoric of choice that operates in the biosocial discourse that surrounds BRCA risk, as their one-size-fits-all nature, plus the nondirective manner in which they must be communicated, create a situation in which each BRCA+ woman must decide which recommendations make sense for her in relation to her personal preferences and family history.

BRCA1 and BRCA2 as "Chromosomal Custodians"

All humans have two copies of the BRCA1 and BRCA2 genes, which are mapped to chromosome 17q and chromosome 13q, respectively. Researchers have long known that the proteins produced by these genes act as tumor suppressors, but the exact nature of their tumor-suppressing function has been unclear. In his contribution to a 2014 special issue of *Science* devoted to breast cancer, Ashok R. Venkitaraman offered the metaphor of "chromosomal custodians" as a way of shedding light on this function, explaining that during the cell cycle BRCA1 and BRCA2 proteins help control the "assembly and activity of macromolecular complexes that monitor chromosome duplication, maintenance, and segregation" (1470). Elaborating precisely what kinds of control BRCA proteins provide is no easy matter, according to Venkitaraman, since they appear to be part of a small subset of proteins that serve as "dynamic hubs" for a number of macromolecular complexes that affect many intracellular components and structures (1470). In other words, it's hard to pinpoint exactly what BRCA proteins do to suppress the development of tumors since they do so much. But by calling them "chromosomal custodians," Venkitaraman means to suggest a specific function for these genes, namely that of preserving the structural and numerical integrity of chromosomes during the cell cycle. Preserving the structural function of chromosomes is largely a matter of repairing the double-strand DNA breaks that can happen as a result of stalled replication forks during chromosome duplication,[4] while preserving the numerical integrity of chromosomes means protecting against aneuploidy during chromosome segregation, or the point in the cell cycle when two sister chromatids separate and move to opposite poles to become new chromosomes (1471–1473).

Both kinds of instability, structural and numerical, accelerate the process of variation and selection that drives carcinogenesis, creating what Venkitaraman describes as a "field of cells susceptible for transformation" (1473). Why this susceptibility manifests more often in BRCA mutation carriers as breast cancer and ovarian cancer is not clear.[5] Venkitaraman offers a few possibilities, for instance, that the tissue-specific functions of breasts and ovaries affect gene expression, that BRCA disruption renders cells in these tissues more sensitive to the effects of local mutagens and rapid cell division, or that these particular tissues allow for the prolonged survival of BRCA deficient cells (1474). What is clear, however, is that when BRCA-related cancers do develop, they and the mutation carriers who get them tend to share a set of common features. For instance, BRCA-related cancers develop more quickly than sporadic cancers, with up to 80 percent of BRCA-related diagnoses occurring in premenopausal women (Pollock and Welsh 86). In addition, contralateral breast cancers and male breast cancers are more common among BRCA mutation carriers compared to noncarriers. As for the cancers themselves, breast cancers in BRCA1 mutation carriers are more likely to be both high grade, meaning their cells are poorly differentiated and have a high rate of mitotic activity, and triple negative, meaning they lack the estrogen receptors, progesterone receptors, and HER2 overexpression that characterize many sporadic breast cancers. Breast cancers in BRCA2 mutation carriers, on the other hand, are more likely to be estrogen receptor positive, even more so than sporadic breast cancers (Pollock and Welsh 86). BRCA-related ovarian cancers are usually high-grade serous tumors that start in the fallopian tubes and spread quickly, a fact that helps to explain why most BRCA+ women who get ovarian cancer are diagnosed at a late stage.

It's important to point out that BRCA mutations are not the only ones that have been linked to higher lifetime risk of breast and ovarian cancers. Mutations in the PALB2, TP53, PTEN, STK11, and CDH1 genes, among others, confer increased risk for developing one or both of these cancers. These mutations, though, have lower penetrance than BRCA mutations, meaning fewer people who carry them will actually develop breast or ovarian cancer. Experts do not agree on exactly how penetrant BRCA mutations are, and more and more research is being done to specify how certain mutation features (e.g., location in the gene and type of nucleotide alteration) affect a carrier's chances of developing cancer.[6] For now, though, most estimates put lifetime breast cancer risk at 50 percent to 80 percent for BRCA1 mutation carriers and 40 to 70 percent for BRCA2 mutation carriers. Lifetime ovarian cancer risks are somewhat lower, an estimated 24 to 40 percent for BRCA1 carriers and 11 to 18 percent for BRCA2 carriers (Petrucelli). Not surprisingly, BRCA+ women are often frustrated by the imprecision of these ranges. A 40 percent lifetime risk of developing breast cancer is very different from an 80 percent risk, and knowing exactly (or even roughly) where one fell between those two numbers could mitigate a great deal of the difficulty surrounding treatment decisions. As it stands, though, most women cannot get more precise risk estimates, and so they are left to consider factors like their own family history and personal preferences when deciding what to do in order to manage their cancer risk. According to the National Comprehensive Cancer Network (NCCN), a consortium of twenty-seven leading cancer treatment and research centers, they should do the following:

+ Begin breast awareness at age eighteen
+ Have clinical breast exams every six to twelve months beginning at age twenty-five
+ Have annual breast MRI (or mammogram if MRI is not available) between ages twenty-five and twenty-nine
+ Have annual breast MRI *and* mammogram between ages thirty and seventy-five
+ Consider risk-reducing bilateral mastectomy
+ Have risk-reducing bilateral salpingo-oophorectomy, typically between ages thirty-five and forty for BRCA1 carriers and between ages forty and forty-five for BRCA2 carriers, and upon completion of child bearing[7]

Of course the operative word in the sentence above is "should." The NCCN recommendations are just that—*recommendations*. As highly penetrant as BRCA mutations can be, no one with a faulty BRCA1 or BRCA2 gene is guaranteed to get cancer. In fact, many BRCA mutation carriers will not develop cancer, despite the fact that family members with the exact same mutations will get the disease. Researchers do not understand why this is the case, but until they do, and until they can use that understanding to refine risk estimates for individual BRCA mutation carriers, then a set of one-size-fits-all management recommendations is the best an organization like the NCCN can do. Simply put, no one can tell a BRCA+ woman that in order to live a long, healthy life, she must make a particular choice about cancer screening or risk-reducing surgeries.[8] And even if they could, that kind of directive would be anathema to the nondirective ethos and ethics that characterize the new genetics and, according to some, protect it from repeating eugenic abuses of the past.[9] Even though the efficacy and desirability of nondirectiveness have been debated for decades in bioethics and genetic counseling, the basic idea that it promotes—namely that patients must be allowed to make their own autonomous decisions about testing and treatment for genetic diseases and susceptibilities—looms large within the biosocial discourses surrounding BRCA risk, fostering a rhetoric of choice that is nothing less than pervasive. No phrase is uttered more frequently in these discourses than "it's your personal choice." As we will see in chapter 2, a great deal of critical ink has been spilled in a decades-long effort to show why this is not the case—why, that is, those at genetic risk are not free to choose, no matter how frequently or fervently they are told otherwise. For the time being, I want to put that debate aside, using the remainder of this chapter to describe the rhetoric of choice that operates within BRCA-related biosocial discourses. To do that, I will sketch its basic contours, focusing on three main components (a rhetoric of autonomous decision making, a rhetoric of nondirectiveness, and a rhetoric of empowerment through knowledge) and showing how they align in key ways with the civic version of the logic of choice as described by Mol. To illustrate these features, I turn to discourse from the FORCE message boards and interviews with BRCA+ women[10] but rely most heavily on examples from three popular BRCA guidebooks: (1) *Confronting Hereditary Breast and Ovarian Cancer: Identify Your Risk, Understand Your Options, Change Your Destiny* (Friedman et al.); (2) *Previvors: Facing the Breast Cancer Gene and Making Life-Changing Decisions* (Port); and (3) *Positive Results: Making the Best Decisions When You're at High Risk for Breast or Ovarian Cancer* (Morris and Gordon). While the universe of BRCA-related biosocial discourse is much wider than this one genre, I have focused on guidebooks because they are a kind of composite genre, one that brings together elements of many genres related to BRCA risk, for example, illness narrative, medical textbook, op-ed, decision guide, and self-help book, among others. Of course, guidebooks are a composite genre that represents very mainstream views on BRCA risk, but that is, in essence, the point—to introduce readers to the mainstream rhetoric of choice that surrounds BRCA risk.

The Rhetoric of Choice in the Biosocial Discourses Surrounding BRCA Risk

When I say that rhetorical appeals to choice in BRCA-related biosocial discourse are pervasive, I mean both that they are made frequently (often multiple times in the same text or section of text), and that they are everywhere, showing up in genres ranging from op-eds, memoirs, and news articles to health promotional materials, product ads, and online message boards. In addition to being pervasive, these appeals are also very predictable insofar as they echo the broader rhetoric of choice that we have come to identify with biomedicine in general and genetic medicine in particular. When it comes to testing and treatment for genetic susceptibility to cancer, BRCA+ women are repeatedly told (and repeatedly tell others) that there are no right or wrong choices, only those that work with their individual situations and those that don't. Readers of *Positive Results*, for instance, are implored to "remember that what may be the right decision for one woman may not be for another. The 'right' decision is the one that fits your life, your circumstances, and your risk tolerance level" (Morris and Gordon 331). This message is echoed in *Previvors*, which reminds readers that while that doctors, friends, and family can try to help a BRCA+ woman figure out this "fit" between her life and her medical decisions, they cannot and should not make the decisions for her (Port 87). "Ultimately, the only opinion that matters is yours," the book advises (119). Medical experts can and should weigh in, but they should not "heavily influence" a woman's decisions about BRCA risk (119). Often invoking the "your body, your choice" rhetoric of the women's health movement, these BRCA guidebooks promote autonomous decision making as the key to empowerment in a situation that is full of potential for disempowerment (119). No woman can control whether or not she inherits a BRCA1 or BRCA2 mutation; nor can she do anything about the limited options available for reducing the cancer risk conferred by those mutations. But she can be the one who chooses among those options, deciding—for herself—what she is or is not willing to do in order to manage or reduce her cancer risk.

This (liberal) feminist message about autonomous decision making reverberates throughout the FORCE message boards, where thousands of women turn for support and advice about how to make those tough decisions about managing or reducing cancer risk. No question is too big or too small for consideration in these boards, and most generate a good deal of discussion, as women at different stages of the "BRCA experience" chime in to share their opinions and advice in order to help others decide which paths to take. Accompanying this willingness to share, however, is a widespread reluctance to come across as too directive or domineering. Thus, there is a great deal of disclaiming in the FORCE message boards, a great deal, that is, of qualifying one's advice with caveats like "whatever you decide is a good decision" or "you have to do what feels right to you." In response to a post about how to time PBM and PBSO, for instance, one woman explained that she decided to have a PBM first and to postpone the PBSO until she was closer to natural menopause. But she cautioned that her decision was also based on her family history (more breast than ovarian cancer) and the fact she was a BRCA2 mutation carrier rather than a BRCA1 mutation carrier. "The decisions are difficult, and require a combination of research, logic, and gut," she wrote. "In the end, there won't be a right decision, but only a best decision, and the best decision will be the one you believe in." A contributor to a thread about having PBSO with or without total hysterectomy couched her advice within a similar proviso, explaining that she chose total hysterectomy because it felt right in her "gut" and made sense in light of her personal preferences and circumstances, for instance, the fact that she felt capable of dealing with the longer recovery time of hysterectomy and that she didn't believe concerns about bladder prolapse after hysterectomy were well founded. "The thing to remember," she advised, "is there is no correct answer; no one should make you feel pressured to do one vs. the other, and no one should make you feel bad for choosing one vs. the other. It's important that we support each other, and you surround yourself with people that support the choices you make." While both of these examples deal with decisions about risk-reducing surgery, this effort to be nondirective extends across the wide range of decision-making situations addressed in the FORCE boards. Whether the question is about how to time yearly mammograms and breast MRIs, the risks and benefits of nipple-sparing mastectomy, or the effectiveness of tamoxifen as a form of chemoprevention, the answer is more often than not some version of "This is what I did, but you should do what's right for you."

If we were to take these elements of the rhetoric of choice at face value, then the message that we would take away from both the guidebooks and the message boards is that all possible choices surrounding BRCA risk testing and treatment are equally valid as long as they are freely chosen. In this sense, the rhetoric of choice here parallels very closely the civic version of the logic of choice described by Mol. As I explained earlier, within this logic, patients are citizens endowed with the right to choose freely, and this right, which is seen as a protection against coercion and oppression, comes before everything else. Mol describes this priority given to choice as an explicit, first level of normativity, explaining that within the civic version of the logic of choice, patients should be able to choose because that gives them autonomy and protects them from coercion. But because of this first layer of normativity, there is a second, implicit layer, one that says the logic of choice should avoid making normative judgments (Mol, *The Logic of Care* 74). Put differently, we could say that because this logic explicitly values choice, it must also implicitly value not making normative judgments about what treatments, goals, or paths are best. Thus, patients are left (even required) to attach their own value to everything *except* their right to choose freely (74). Within this logic and according to these layers of normativity, it makes perfect sense to say, as one FORCE contributor did in response to a BRCA1 mutation carrier's question about pregnancy and PBM, that "whatever you decide is a good decision." The implication here is not just that the BRCA1 mutation carrier will make the right decision but also (and more so) that the decision will be right *because she will have been the one to have made it.*

While choosing freely is indeed the most important activity according to this rhetoric of choice, it is not one that just any BRCA+ woman can participate in. That's not to say that choosing freely is something reserved for only a select few, or even that it has to be earned necessarily, but rather that it is typically framed as the outcome of an educational process, one that requires a woman to not just face the facts about BRCA risk but to seek them out, gathering as much knowledge as possible and then carefully evaluating it from the perspective of their personal preferences. Within this context knowledge is something BRCA+ women are "armed" with (Port 57), something that is "both empowering and comforting" (Friedman et al. xix), and something that allows them to "avoid being victimized" (Morris and Gordon 13). Such characterizations were commonly used by the BRCA+ women I interviewed, especially Gina, a twenty-eight-year-old from Nebraska, and Cheri, a twenty-three-year-old from Texas. When I asked Gina what it was like to live with a BRCA mutation, she said that she felt "lucky or blessed" because knowing about her mutation meant she had a choice in treatment, that she could do preventative surgery if she wanted or use screening to catch cancer early if she opted against it. Of course, this didn't mean that she was "excited" to have a BRCA mutation, but compared to "women just walking about their day" for whom a cancer diagnosis might be a surprise, Gina felt like her knowledge gave her an edge, that it made her better prepared for what might lie ahead. Cheri's feelings of gratitude and optimism were expressed in even stronger terms. She told me that knowing about her mutation was one of the "most empowering experiences" of her life. Having watched her mother die of breast cancer at a young age, Cheri perceived her recent PBM as a way to "stop cancer in its tracks." "Sometimes I feel like my mom had to lose her battle so that my siblings and I could win the war against cancer by preventing it altogether," she explained. Overall, Cheri felt empowered not only by knowledge of her genetic mutation but also by the chance to share her story and show other families that "these cancers don't have to be a death sentence."

By portraying knowledge in these terms, as a precondition of autonomy and empowerment, this rhetoric of choice again corresponds closely with the civic version of the logic of choice: within both, choosing freely is a right but one that brings with it a responsibility to know and weigh all the relevant facts. While all of the guidebooks try to help BRCA+ women fulfill this responsibility, none do so as clearly and schematically as *Confronting Hereditary Breast and Ovarian Cancer*, the BRCA guidebook officially endorsed by FORCE and co-authored by FORCE founder Sue Friedman. There, in the final chapter, "Putting the Pieces Together to Make Difficult Decisions," readers are told that making decisions related to BRCA risk "can be agonizing," but that by knowing all of their options and relying on "credible and up-to-date information," they will be able to consider each option and make the choices that are best for them (228–29). To facilitate this decision-making process, this chapter includes a table, "Comparing Risk-Reducing Alternatives," that lists each possible action a BRCA+ woman might take (e.g., doing breast surveillance), the benefit it provides (e.g., increases odds of finding cancer early), and limitations or risks it entails (e.g., does not prevent cancer) (232). Readers are advised that to use the table, they should work their way through each option, listing additional advantages and disadvantages that will affect them personally, eliminating the unacceptable actions, and then prioritizing those that remain (231–33). Although the authors of *Confronting Hereditary Breast and Ovarian Cancer* try to be careful about not oversimplifying decisions surrounding BRCA risk, the message here is clear: if you empower yourself with knowledge, then you might not be able to have what you want, but you can be the one who chooses from among the available options.

I could go on here, providing additional examples from these guidebooks and message boards, as well as other BRCA-related texts, but if the goal is to introduce readers to this rhetoric of choice, then I am not convinced those examples would tell us anything new. In some sense, what needs to be said has been said before—and much of it by Mol in her description of the civic version of the logic of choice. Rhetoric and logic are not the same thing, of course, but the truth is that a great deal of what BRCA+ women say about their experience (and a great deal of what is said on their behalf) aligns with key features Mol attributes to that logic, especially the unwillingness to make normative judgments about anything *except* the right to choose freely and the emphasis on knowledge as key to empowerment. There is, however, another feature that Mol attributes to this logic of choice, one that I didn't describe earlier but that I want to turn to now, before drawing this chapter to a close. Near the end of *The Logic of Care*, Mol compares "styles of judgment" within the two versions of the logic choice, arguing that while customers choose individually and privately, citizens "rule together," coordinating their personal choices in public through "conversations about what it might be good to do" (74–75). We can see this "style of judgment" on display in a number of the genres that populate the universe of BRCA-related biosocial discourse but in none so clearly as the FORCE message boards, where women turn to ask questions, seek advice and support, and vet ideas or treatment plans. While I am not prepared to claim here that these message boards reveal any new features of the rhetoric of choice (though a deeper investigation might very well produce such insight), I do think they can help us to understand its staying power and value. Earlier I suggested that this staying power is tied to the need to separate the new genetics from eugenics, that is, to show that by making a patient's participation in genetic medicine a matter of personal choice, we are not repeating the grave ethical and political mistakes of the past. I still believe this is the case, that what happens at broader levels of ethics and biopolitics is picked up and cycled through the discourses of BRCA+ women.[11] But I also believe that the staying power and value of this rhetoric are tied to this "style of judgment," as Mol puts it, and what it allows BRCA+ women as health-care citizens to do: deliberate collectively to determine what they will and will not do to their bodies, families, and lives in order to manage or reduce their cancer risk. By tacking a phrase like "but it's your personal choice" or "whatever you decide is the right decision" on to a piece of advice or an anecdote, no woman is actually guaranteeing another's ability to choose freely. This is not a situation in which saying it's so makes it so. But that woman is, I think, making it easier to share the specifics of her own experiences, to explain in detail what went well or not so well with a certain procedure or practice. Such detail is incredibly important in these decision-making situations, and I think those clichéd phrases about making personal choices that fit individual circumstances and preferences can act as a kind of permission slip for providing it, for offering one's personal experience about such high-stakes issues and questions. In this sense, then, we might think of this rhetoric of choice as a series of beau gestes, that is, as a set of predictable but also well-meaning and perhaps even noble gestures that are important in form but almost entirely meaningless in substance. Their meaninglessness—that is, the fact that they do not guarantee anyone's ability to choose freely and might even diminish it—is the subject of chapter 2, to which I now turn.

2

From Ideology to Governmentality | A Constructivist
View of Genetic Risk

Kelly Happe frames her 2013 book, *The Material Gene: Gender, Race, and Hered-ity After the Human Genome Project* with a very provocative question: "How do we think of heredity and disease not as recalcitrant material realities discovered by researchers and physicians but as contingent manifestations of the lived social experience of worlds?" (2). Her aim, which this question makes clear, is to cut the Gordian knot, as Latour would put it. We can understand heredity and disease either in terms of nature, that is, as "recalcitrant material realities," or in terms of culture, that is, as "the lived experience of social worlds," but not in terms of both. Thus, we must choose, and in choosing we must purify one from the other. According to Latour, this act of purification is the hallmark of moder-nity (Latour, *We Have Never Been Modern* 10–11). It constantly creates hybrids or quasi-objects—things that are not ontologically pure, not reducible to either the human realm or the nonhuman realm—and then assigns itself the task of purifying them, of either "bracketing all dogma and occult properties to arrive at a theory of nature in itself, or by turning a skeptical glance toward all scientific claims so as to view them as the surface effects of human political and linguistic convention" (Harman, *Towards Speculative Realism* 76). What struck me about Happe's question the first time I read it is the implication that engaging in this form of purification would mean going against the grain, as though the audience would have to be won over to an unfamiliar way of thinking. Indeed, my second reaction to the question was to pose another: How can we think of heredity and disease as something *other* than cultural constructions? What resources do we have within the social sciences and humanities for understanding the reality of heredity and disease without sliding back into a kind of naïve realism that would enact the very same form of purification, only in the opposite direction? The point of the next chapter is to answer that question. The point of this chap-ter is to demonstrate that we need to. The constructivist paradigm has domi-nated scholarship on risk in the social sciences and humanities for decades, exposing the human motives and discursive forces operating behind the illusion of nature. And there's no question that this has been an important undertaking, especially in the case of genetic risk, where the specter of genetic determinism always looms.[1] As long as we view genetic risk as a construction, and, as long as we continually reveal how that construction works, then we have some measure of protection against the very dangerous idea that our health can be reduced to the function of our genes. As history has shown us this idea comes with a very high price tag.

But at this point—a point when there are good reasons for rejecting the idea that contemporary genetic medicine is simply the newest incarnation of eugenics[2]—I believe that a continued commitment to constructivism comes with a cost as well. This cost is the subject of Latour's "Why Has Critique Run Out of Steam?: From Matters of Fact to Matters of Concern," the well-known 2004 essay where he indicts the modern critical stance for its ceaseless repetition of a set of constructivist moves that has not only failed to achieve the amelioration it aimed for but has also prevented us from revising our critical approaches to better suit present challenges (231). The specific problem for Latour is that constructivism has just two ways of dealing with hybrid objects. On the one hand, it locates them at the "fairy position," which is used by social scientists engaged in a kind of anti-fetishism; the aim here "is to show that what the naïve believers are doing with objects is simply a projection of their wishes onto a material entity that does nothing at all by itself" (237). In other words, no matter what idol some group believes in—god, sports, art, and so forth—the aim is to show that its power is not innate but rather comes from them, from society. On the other hand, there's the "fact position," which corresponds most closely with the kinds of constructivist critiques I'll discuss in this chapter. Here the critic shows the naïve believers that while they might think they are free, they are actually acted on by unforeseen forces, which the critic explains by marshaling whichever "pet facts" she prefers to work with (238). These facts can come from any number of sources—economics, neurobiology, critical theory, wherever. What matters is that their "origin, fabrication, [and] mode of development" go unquestioned while the critic uses them to demonstrate that the believer's freedom is an illusion (238). Often animated by a hermeneutics of suspicion, this kind of critique pivots around an appearance/reality distinction that puts the critic in the role of decoder and debunker. Together Latour sees these two positions, fairy and fact, as a kind of critical double blow. As soon as the first position gives the believers some faith in "their own projective capacity,"

the critic hits them with a "second uppercut," humiliating them by demonstrating that no matter what they think, "their behavior is entirely determined by
the action of powerful causalities coming from an objective reality they don't
see, but that you, yes you, the never sleeping critic, alone can see" (239). No
matter how these blows are administered, the outcome is the same: science and
society are purified from one another and anyone caught believing in the reality
of an object is determined to be incredibly naïve (Latour, *We Have Never Been
Modern* 6).

Admittedly, Latour's punching metaphor is a bit hyperbolic, and I am not
suggesting that critics of genetic risk are out to humiliate the "naïve believers."
Yet I think Latour's point still has a great deal of merit, especially in the case of
genetic risk, which is about as hybrid an object as any that science and society
have ever produced. Yet when we operate within a constructivist paradigm, our
job is to ignore this hybridity, turning a skeptical eye not only toward science but
also toward those who trust science and believe that there is something real
about genetic risk. More often than not, this means that their discourses—and
the medical and scientific discourses they draw on—are interpreted as indices
and/or sources of ideological mystification, that is, evidence of how they've been
manipulated and how they, wittingly or not, are manipulating others. Taking on
the role of debunker, we then attempt to explain how they have been tricked,
presumably on the assumption that they would choose differently if they knew
differently. As I intimated in the introduction, however, this assumption is
fraught with problems, not the least of which is its inability to account for the
fact that individuals can recognize a behavior as ideological and yet continue
participating in it anyway. Thus, with Latour, I would argue that it is time to
retool, time, that is, to cultivate ways of critically engaging the ethics, politics,
and rhetorics of the new genetics that aim to do something other than enlighten
the naïve believers. This, of course, is what I hope to achieve through a rhetoric
of care.

As an initial step toward this goal, this chapter reviews constructivist critiques of genetic risk and the rhetorics of choice that have developed around
them. Specifically, it argues that these critiques are organized—either explicitly
or implicitly—around one of two key concepts: ideology or governmentality. In
the case of the former, the argument is very familiar; indeed it corresponds very
closely to the one I outlined above. Critics typically claim that genetic science
and medicine serve an ideological function by naturalizing dominant ideas
about race, gender, and class and then seek to explain how various discourses

mask this function. Again, because I indicated the problems with this kind of ideology critique in the introduction, I do not want to rehash them here. It is worth noting, however, that it illustrates precisely Latour's problem with the "fact position" insofar as the only thing to which it grants any reality are those hidden ideological forces. Thus, even in critiques that adopt very strong constructivist positions, arguing that since everything is the product of discursive forces, there is no chance of seeing things as they "really are," the analysis still tends to pivot around an appearance/reality distinction that positions the critic as decoder and debunker.[3] In theory, analyses of genetic risk based on the concept of governmentality should avoid this problem, and some do.[4] As I will explain later, governmentality studies seek to understand how government works as the "conduct of conduct" or, more specifically, how it produces free subjects who, by choosing to participate in certain practices or techniques of the self, serve the ends of the government while also serving themselves (Rose et al. 89). What makes this framework a more appealing option for critics who want to avoid the problems of ideology critique is that by not acknowledging a polarity between freedom and domination, it is able to shift attention from questions about *why* or in whose interests government operates to questions about *how* it operates (Rose et al. 93). Yet because governmentality-based critiques of genetic risk tend to take strong constructivist positions on the nature of risk, questions about hidden purposes reemerge, placing hybrid objects like genetic risk in the fact position just as much as ideology critique. In the specific case of breast and ovarian cancer risk, this combination typically produces critiques that, despite their increased focus on what genetically at-risk women actually *do* in order to prevent cancer, consistently return to the idea that exposing the ideological function of these practices will make those women free to choose differently.

There would be no way, within the space of this chapter, to review all of the work on genetic risk that has employed these two concepts; thus, the review I offer here is selective, aiming to show the development of common lines of argument and structures of explanation within these two categories of constructivist critiques of risk. In the first half of the chapter, I focus on ideology, reviewing a number of early critiques that warned of the oppressive, eugenic ideologies operating within genetic science and medicine. I then turn to the argument about hereditarian ideology and BRCA mutations that Happe makes in chapter 3 of *The Material Gene*, "Genomics and the Reproductive Body." I focus on Happe's argument here not only because it demonstrates how ingrained and repetitive the moves of ideology critique have become by 2013 but also what they yield in the particular context of genetic risk for breast and ovarian cancers. The second half of the chapter unfolds somewhat differently. Here, I illustrate how the concept of governmentality has been used to understand genetic risk for breast and ovarian cancers by reviewing four studies, two of cancer diagnostic practices and two of cancer prevention practices. However, I do more to contextualize those arguments, beginning with a description of the concept of governmentality and then moving to an explanation of where and how it has merged with constructivist views of risk to produce a kind of critique that still pivots around the appearance/reality distinction so central to ideology critique. It is important to note here, as I do again in the conclusion, that by setting up this work on genetic risk as the problem, which is to say, as the tradition we need to move away from, I do not mean to suggest that the insights it has produced are wrong.[5] There would be something deeply ironic about taking issue with a set of arguments that pivot around an appearance/reality distinction by trying to show where they went wrong or how they mask the truth of genetic risk. Moreover, it would be naïve to deny the political function of genetic risk, whether that function is understood in terms of ideology, governmentality, or both. Yet it would also be naïve, I think, to think to just dig in our heels and trust that if we keep exposing this function, it will go away.

Genetic Risk and/as Ideology

In their 1984 *Not in Our Genes: Biology, Ideology, and Human Nature*, Richard Lewontin, Steven Rose, and Leon Kamin compared their job as critics of biological determinism to that of a fire brigade whose members were constantly being called out in the middle of the night to put out one "conflagration" after another. "Now it's IQ and race, now criminal genes, now the biological inferiority of women, now the genetic fixity of human nature." All of these "deterministic fires" need to be doused with the "cold water of reason," they argued, before the "entire intellectual neighborhood" goes up in flames (265). Descriptions of these "deterministic fires" and warnings about their increasing frequency set the stage for dozens of critiques of genetic science and medicine in the 1980s and 1990s. Often citing the media's obsessive coverage of "discoveries" like the "gay gene," the "violence gene," and the "addiction gene," critics cautioned that biological explanations of human health, behavior, and identity were making a comeback; and they almost always framed this comeback within the same historical narrative:

the rise of eugenics in the early twentieth century; its demise after the atrocities of Nazi eugenic policy in WWII; the triumph of nurture over nature in the 1950s and 1960s; and then a slow but steady return of biological determinism beginning in the 1970s and reaching its apex and most obvious manifestation in the 1990 establishment of the HGP. Many critics saw this return of biological explanations as a conservative backlash against social welfare policies and the civil and women's rights movements, arguing that even if the new genetics focused on the health of individuals rather than the health of the gene pool, its discriminatory origins and potential were just as threatening as that of the eugenics movement. In fact, some worried that since this version of biological determinism operated under the protective cover of scientific objectivity and medical beneficence, it posed an even greater threat.

The concept of ideology was, in many ways, the perfect tool for explaining this hidden threat. According to its basic definition, ideology refers to something illusory, usually a set of ideas or practices that mask or invert reality, thus allowing one group to dominate another.[6] What's key about this domination, though, is that it doesn't require force. On account of the illusions perpetuated by ideology, dominated groups participate willingly in their domination. In other words, they are complicit in their own exploitation, and it's not until they are made aware of this fact through ideology critique that progress can be achieved. Thus, the task of the critic is to identify the contradictions that ideology has masked over. This understanding of ideology is, indeed, quite basic, but it is the one that has most consistently been deployed in critiques of genetic science and medicine and the rhetorics of choice they promote. Some critics have executed this task of unmasking contradictions from an explicitly Marxist perspective, arguing that biological determinism is a way of legitimizing economic inequalities in industrialized capitalist societies. This was the primary claim of both Lewontin, Rose, and Kamin's *Not in Our Genes* and Lewontin's subsequent *Biology as Ideology: The Doctrine of DNA*. Focusing on the supposed genetic basis of things like mental illness, intelligence, patriarchy, and criminal violence, both of these books sought to expose the mutually reinforcing relationship between bourgeois social values and reductionist scientific principles. Lewontin extended this Marxist critique in *Biology as Ideology*, arguing that science was inevitably ideological because it used commodities and was part of the process of commodity production (4). By confusing heredity for fixity, he argued, biological determinism is the "most powerful single weapon that biological ideologues have had in legitimating a society of inequality," and, since biologists should know better, that is, since they should know that DNA does not unilaterally determine life, we must at least suspect that they are "beneficiaries" of these inequalities and, as a result, cannot be trusted as "objective experts" (37).

Other critics were less Marxist in their understanding of ideology, but the general aim of their argument—to reveal the eugenic threat operating beneath the veneer of scientific objectivity—was the same. In *Backdoor to Eugenics*, for example, Troy Duster claimed that no matter how well intentioned scientists' motives appeared to be, an orientation toward genetic susceptibility couldn't help but to dominate and distort our ways of thinking about disease prevention (123). Duster used the metaphor of a "prism of heritability" to describe this process, arguing that once a disorder is understood as genetic, only two modes of prevention appear possible: altering the affected genes or setting up genetic screening programs (55). Both solutions threatened to open a "backdoor" to eugenics, he argued, but we fail to recognize this threat because it's obscured by a discourse of scientific, health, and medical benefits (129). Efforts to screen workers for genetic susceptibility to chronic lung disease, for instance, might seem like a reasonable way to reduce suffering, but in reality those efforts bear a hidden message, namely that it's better to exclude certain types of people from certain types of jobs than it is to clean up the workplace (123). Duster called for a critical examination of these "hidden arguments" or "subterranean political ideologies," arguing that it would take a vigorous public debate and an informed public policy to stem the tide of biological determinism (113, 129).

Abby Lippmann shared Duster's concerns, but in her view, the idea of a "prism of heritability" didn't go far enough to explain the problem. Genetics is not just a prism through which knowledge can be refracted, she argued, but is instead the "source of the illumination itself" ("Prenatal Testing and Screening" 19). Thus, Lippmann coined a new term, "geneticization," which she defined as the ideology and the practice "by which differences between individuals are reduced to their DNA codes, with most disorders, behaviors, and psychological variations defined, at least in part, as genetic in origin" (19).[7] Lippman's work focused specifically on geneticization within the context of prenatal diagnostics, as she sought to expose the eugenic reality operating beneath the rhetoric of autonomy, choice, and reassurance used to market genetic testing to pregnant women (23–25). Eugenic intent is regularly denied in biomedical reports about prenatal diagnosis, she maintained, but such denials are "disingenuous" since no matter how else we choose to define it, prenatal genetic testing and screening "*is* a means of separating fetuses we wish to develop from those we wish to discontinue" (23). And making it a matter of "choice" does not change this fact. In a line of reasoning that would be repeated and developed by many after her, Lippman argued that real choice cannot exist in a society that does little to accommodate the needs of disabled children (32) and that makes the women who give birth to them feel guilty and inadequate for not ensuring a better pregnancy outcome (28).

Lippman's notion of geneticization had a wide impact outside the context of prenatal diagnostics, in part, no doubt, because it so succinctly summarized the case against genetic medicine. In this sense, it functioned much like the earlier term, "medicalization," implying the unwarranted and ethically dangerous movement of biomedical authority into facets of human experience previously understood in nonbiomedical terms (Illich; Ten Have). Some critics studied this movement within the context of specific diseases in order to identify the scientific and social mechanisms by which a genetic disease definition replaced a nongenetic one. Hoedemaekers and Ten Have's 1998 study, "Geneticization: The Cyprus Paradigm," is representative in this regard. Focusing on beta thalassemia prevention policy in Cyprus in the 1970s and 1980s, they explained how health professionals encouraged the adoption of a genetic approach to the disease and how this adoption, in turn, resulted in certain "incongruities" between appearance and reality, for example, the fact that genetic screening was promoted on the basis of free choice but executed within a directive environment and, relatedly, that advocates of screening denied eugenic intent while simultaneously promoting its economic benefits for the community and the state (282, 284). Another 1998 study, this time on the geneticization of breast cancer, also illustrates well the utility of Lippman's argument. In "Breast Cancer: Reading the Omens," Margaret Lock argued that the then-new technology of genetic testing for breast cancer susceptibility encouraged a biologically reductivist style of reasoning, one that eclipsed a better understanding of the environmental causes of the disease and created not just "heightened anxiety" but also a "moral discourse" about prevention that made health an individual responsibility (8, 10).

Other studies aimed for a broader critique of geneticization, focusing on either the faulty science behind it or its effects within popular culture. In *Exploding the Gene Myth*, for example, Ruth Hubbard and Elijah Wald argued that the "various ideological roots" of genetics are difficult to identity because the public has been conditioned to accept the idea that "the march of science is immune from political and societal pressures" (7). Specifically, they sought to dispel the dangerous and misleading idea that genotype and phenotype exist in a relationship of one-to-one correspondence. To this end, they debunked the popularly held belief that a single gene "codes for" a single protein, explaining that in order for any protein to be synthesized, a cell's "entire metabolic apparatus," which includes many proteins and, therefore, many genes, must function properly (52). Extending this line of argument throughout their book, Hubbard and Wald challenged the research linking complex, multifactorial disorders like diabetes, high blood pressure, and cancer, as well as traits such as sexual orientation and proclivity to violence, to an individual's genetic makeup. Dorothy Nelkin and Susan Lindee took a similarly broad approach in their 1995 *The DNA Mystique: The Gene as Cultural Icon*, but their goal was to understand how the gene as a symbol served "ideological purposes and institutional agendas" within popular culture, independent of its biological definitions (5, 16). Thus, theirs was a task of decoding slogans, ads, newspaper and magazine articles, TV shows, movies, jokes, and cartoons in order to demonstrate how the gene was used to not only define identity, relationships, and health but also to assign guilt and responsibility, to protect power and privilege, and to judge the morality of social systems. Jose van Dijk took on a similar task in her 1998 *Imagenation: Population Images of Genetics*, explaining how popular representations of genetics are shaped by ideological forces that affect our understanding of scientific purpose and progress.

As I said at the outset, this review is selective, but something more comprehensive would only belabor a point that is already obvious: since the 1980s, critiques of genetic science and medicine that employ the concept of ideology have focused on a variety of objects, but the structure of the explanations they provide has been remarkably consistent. Whether or not ideology is actually defined, exposing its operation is a matter of distinguishing reality from appearance, a matter, that is, of showing how something that appears natural, objective, and beneficent is actually constructed, motivated, and oppressive. Happe's 2013 *The Material Gene* very much continues in this tradition; in fact, in many ways its overarching aim is to refute those who have tried to challenge the easy identification of the new genetics with eugenics. Nikolas Rose, for instance, has challenged this identification by arguing that the "style of thinking" within genomics has been "molecularized," which is to say that the object under investigation is no longer a "gene" but rather the mechanical and biological properties that make up a "gene" and regulate its transcription and expression (*Politics of Life Itself* 5–6, 12). For Rose, this shift toward molecularization means that genetic research is moving away from a world of "depths and determinations" and into one of "surfaces and associations," one, that is, where the genetic code is understood as "one set of relays in complex, ramifying, and nonhierarchical networks, filiations, and connections" rather than a "deep structure that causes or determines" (130). On these grounds Rose has repeatedly rejected the idea that the best way to engage and understand the new genetics is to critique it by looking for the hidden motives behind genetic determinism (258). In *The Material Gene*, Happe calls for precisely this kind of critique, arguing that the same "hereditarian ideology" that informed eugenics operates within new genetics, bringing with it "a concomitant regressive politics" that attributes "the causes of material and social inequalities to the pathologies of particular bodies" (4, 23–24). In her view, in fact, eugenics was an early example of this "explanatory capacity," and today, despite efforts to "revise itself" after the eugenic movement, contemporary genetics has not been able to abandon "its investment in the normalization of bodies and the larger social and economic order" (5).

However, this investment has become harder to identify, as it has moved into what Happe, following Fredric Jameson and Sandra Harding, calls the "political unconscious" of science's "cognitive core." There it lies hidden, operating under the mystifying cover of not just institutional discourses of medicine, health, and healing, as critics like Duster and Lippman argued, but also beneath recent scientific developments (e.g., the turn to epigenetics noted by Rose) and political movements (e.g., feminism and environmentalism) that have "compelled significant discursive shifts" but done little to challenge biomedicine's production of a "particular, gendered, racialized, economic order" (12–14). To expose this contradiction, Happe employs a rhetorical methodology, one that focuses on how the "material exigencies and constraints" of a particular institutional discourse, along with "particular tropes, arguments, and linguistic arrangements" together constitute "its meaning-making practices" (17). Such an approach is warranted, she argues, not only because discourse is the means by which dominant ideas are circulated, but also because the objects of study here—namely the body and genetic risk—are, themselves, discursive productions (14–15, 178).[8]

From this constructivist perspective, Happe works as decoder throughout *The Material Gene*, explaining how these purportedly natural phenomena, the body and the gene, have been "inscribed by the social" in ways that maintain status quo interests (179). Here, I want to focus on her argument in chapter 3, "Genomics and the Reproductive Body," because it offers a clear and, I think, fairly representative example of what this kind of decoding yields in the particular case of BRCA mutations. The specific object of analysis in the chapter is the use of prophylactic bilateral salpingo oophorectomy to prevent ovarian cancer in women with BRCA mutations. Women with diagnosed BRCA mutations are estimated to have a 16.5 to 63 percent lifetime risk of developing ovarian cancer (Petrucelli). PBSO, the prophylactic removal of both ovaries and the fallopian tubes, is seen as a reasonable response to this risk in large part because ovarian cancer is very difficult to detect and treat.[9] Most cases (60 percent) are diagnosed at stage III or later, which means that the cancer has spread beyond the pelvis and the five-year survival rate is approximately 34 percent ("Survival Rates"). Happe questions this justification of the procedure, however, arguing that beneath it lies a "more complicated narrative," one in which the routinization of PBSO for cancer prevention is a "sociopolitical phenomenon" that has as much to do with legitimizing medicine and protecting heterosexist gender norms as it does with preventing a deadly disease (77). To expose this narrative, Happe does two things: first, she historicizes PBSO, showing that the development of the procedure and its acceptance as a cancer prevention strategy cannot be separated from its eugenic past; and second, she analyzes the "conceptual and epistemological significance" of clinical risk assessments in order to distinguish the real function of BRCA testing from its apparent function.

The key claim in Happe's historical narrative is that the prophylactic removal of the ovaries to prevent ovarian cancer for BRCA+ women is but one rationale of ovary removal in a long series of rationales designed to legitimate gynecology as a medical specialization (67). These rationales have always corresponded to social and cultural ideas about femininity and reproduction, and they have often explicitly borne the imprint of eugenics. For instance, Happe explains that in the nineteenth century, doctors argued that oophorectomy was needed to sterilize women "unfit" to reproduce and to cure conditions such as ovarian prolapse, menstrual madness, hysterical vomiting, and nymphomania (68–69). Eventually, critics challenged these arguments, but their counterarguments did nothing to diminish the power of eugenics since they cautioned against ovary removal on the grounds that women needed to reproduce in order to fulfill their function in life and that low reproduction rates from certain kinds of women would result in race suicide (71). In the mid-twentieth century, however, these cultural rationales for oophorectomy began to fall out of favor, and, as a result, physicians and surgeons focused on the threat of ovarian cancer, arguing that once reproduction was complete, ovaries had little use and carried a special proclivity for cancer (71–72). From a positivist perspective, Happe argues, this transition to cancer prevention would seem to signal that gynecology had moved into "a more enlightened period of its history," but in reality it shows that the field continued to serve the same status quo interests by continuing to reduce ovaries to their reproductive function (71, 77).

However, this rationale—that ovaries are dangerous and expendable after reproduction—did not go unchallenged. Indeed, this challenge, which came in the form of studies demonstrating both the risks of oophorectomy and the benefit of ovarian conservation, is a key part of Happe's narrative insofar as it highlights the role of BRCA research in the procedure's ongoing struggle for legitimation. As Happe explains it, by acknowledging the risks of ovary removal and the value of ovarian function, these studies created another legitimacy crisis for oophorectomy. After all, how could the procedure be justified if the benefits of conservation were judged to be greater than the risk of ovarian cancer? The answer is BRCA research, which by exempting a whole population from the recommendation to conserve nondiseased ovaries created "a new constituency for the long embattled procedure" (87). But this development only raises a new, more significant question, namely, how do BRCA mutation carriers gain this exceptional status? That is, how does it become "thinkable" that BRCA mutation carriers would undergo the same medical treatment as ovarian cancer patients (66, 80)?

The short answer to this question is an oft-repeated observation in critiques like Happe's, namely that in the era of the new genetics, risk itself becomes the disease. But Happe's explanation goes further, showing that in the case of BRCA-related cancer risk, this mistake happens because clinical risk assessment, that is, the kind of risk assessment that comes from genetic testing for BRCA mutations, "is taken to be substantially and materially different from family history (and thus constitutes a novel scientific object)" (62). In other words, it "operates as a distinct epistemological category," providing an "indisputable basis for action" (80). Citing several medical research studies, Happe argues that one key reason for this distinction between clinical risk and familial risk—and for the devaluation of the latter in favor of the former—is geneticists' belief that BRCA testing can reduce the uncertainty surrounding a woman's risk status, thus allowing her to make better decisions about prophylactic surgery (79).

Happe mounts several challenges to this reasoning, and I want to review each since they are the basis of her understanding of the "conceptual and epistemological significance" of the BRCA test and, thus, the grounds on which she distinguishes their real function from their apparent function. First Happe notes that "the risk associated with BRCA mutations, much like the concept of risk more generally, is not an objective fact, but a social construct" (79).[10] She then questions the idea that clinical risk assessments are qualitatively different from familial risk assessments on the grounds that "both produce statistical probability statements—[which is to say that] the *telos* of both types of analysis is to establish risk, not diagnose disease" (79). Furthermore, she argues that the information produced by clinical risk assessment is affected by several scientific and technological limitations, namely that it is based on the "presumed function" of an inherited mutation (meaning that scientists do not understand precisely how the addition or deletion of a nucleotide in a mutation affects the function of BRCA1 and BRCA2 genes) and that "data are limited to the study of only some of the thousands of known mutations" (79). And finally, she points out that the special legitimacy granted to clinical risk assessment is related to the privilege that vision-based knowledge holds in medicine. "Implicitly," she argues, "genomics benefits from visual culture insofar as the DNA base pairs of the genetic test allow the diagnostician to 'see' the very thing that increases a woman's risk for cancer [. . .] BRCA tests, we are told, reveal 'actual risk' of 'genetically defined' women" (80). Yet, according to Happe, what exactly distinguishes one's family history from one's genome is nothing more than "a shift in the field of vision" (80).

Based on these limitations, Happe determines that the "conceptual and epistemological significance" of the BRCA test "lies not in how it produces accurate assessments of actually existing risk" but rather in the way it "substitutes the mark of ancestry for the materially lived experience, removing from the clinician's gaze a range of mitigating and aggravating variables that would otherwise influence what counts as actionable risk" (78). In other words, what the BRCA test actually accomplishes is the "conceptual removal of a woman from a particular context or environment and, with that, a consideration of embodied life in all its complexity" (80). And the result of this decontextualization, in turn, is that the "putatively real risk" associated with BRCA mutations makes carriers "unqualified candidates" for prophylactic oophorectomy with one key exception: only those women who want to have children and who are still young enough to do so are told that surveillance, rather than surgery, for ovarian cancer risk is a rational choice (90, 93). Happe argues that this exception is made possible by a set of heterosexist gender norms that, according to the same logic that operated in the earlier rationales for oophorectomy, prioritizes a woman's reproductive capacity and desire over everything else (92). Thus, she concludes that even though "the surface-level justifications for prophylactic oophorectomy may have changed from the treatment of psychic disorders to the reduction of cancer risk, the justificatory logics are similar, as is the impact on women's bodies" (99). In other words, BRCA research "is a recuperative project, both for its own ever-changing institutional needs and for a larger social order threatened by feminist and queer theorizing that destabilizes our unquestioned beliefs about the biological foundations of the sexed and gendered body" (100).

So, here we have the real function of the BRCA test—its cultural function—separated from its apparent function—its scientific function. To explain what's troubling about this separation, I want to call attention to two facts that Happe's argument omits. First, it omits the fact that BRCA mutation carriers who have PBSO *do not* undergo the same medical treatment as the overwhelming majority of ovarian cancer patients. Because most ovarian cancers have spread by the time of diagnosis, debulking surgery is required. The aim of debulking surgery is to remove, in addition to the ovaries and fallopian tubes, as much tumor as possible and any organ or part of an organ that the tumor has invaded, such as the uterus, cervix, pelvic lymph nodes, liver, diaphragm, spleen, or intestines. This brutal surgery, which can have debilitating side effects, is followed by chemotherapy and radiation. It usually results in "suboptimal cytoreduction," which means that visible tumor is left behind, and the chance of recurrence, as well as additional debulking surgery, is extremely high. It would seem that any examination of the factors that make PBSO a "thinkable" option for women at genetic risk of breast and ovarian cancers would need to account for these differences. However, this isn't even the question that Happe asked. Her question—how does it become "thinkable" that women at risk could undergo this same treatment as cancer patients—obscures the differences between PBSO and ovarian cancer treatment, thus creating an even stronger exigence for the kind of ideology critique she provides.

Second, Happe's argument omits the fact that in cases where a BRCA mutation has been identified, clinical risk assessments *do* reduce the uncertainty surrounding a woman's mutation status. BRCA mutations are passed down according to an autosomal dominant pattern of inheritance, which means that the child of a mutation carrier has a 50 percent chance of inheriting her or his parent's mutation and that only one mutated allele is required to produce susceptibility. Thus, on the one hand, if a mutation has been identified in a family with cases of breast and/or ovarian cancer, and a woman tests negative, then she absolutely knows something she did not know before: that she did not inherit the mutation. This knowledge doesn't mean she won't get cancer. But, barring any other mutation or abnormal environmental exposure, her risk is the same as the risk of a noncarrier. On the other hand, if there's a known mutation and a woman tests positive, she too knows something that she did not know before: she did inherit a mutation. As Happe points out, this does not mean that she will develop cancer since BRCA mutations do not have 100 percent penetrance. But regardless, this fact about BRCA testing—that it reveals if a mutation was inherited—greatly affects its "conceptual and epistemological significance"; indeed, this fact, not the idea that it diagnoses "actual risk," marks the primary difference between clinical risk assessments and familial risk assessments. Yet neither it nor the difference between PBSO and ovarian cancer treatment warrant mentioning in Happe's argument. These omissions are evidence, I think, not of why her conclusions about the heterosexist history of PBSO are wrong. Rather, these omissions are evidence of how completely she has tried to purify culture from nature. In Happe's argument, if PBSO is the product of a eugenic, misogynist history (and I believe she makes a convincing case that it is), then that is *all* it can be. Likewise, if BRCA testing provides justification for a procedure that has a eugenic history, then that is *all* it can do. There is no room within such a narrow and thoroughly suspicious perspective for acknowledging that a woman who tests positive for a BRCA mutation can have good reasons for having a PBSO or for postponing one in order to have children. These reasons do not negate the procedure's heterosexist history and effects, but they do matter, and neither they nor the scientific/medical facts on which they might be based—for example, that PBSO and ovarian cancer treatment *are not* the same and that clinical risk assessments *are* different from familial risk assessments—should be swallowed up by the interpretive apparatus of a constructivist paradigm that reduces everything to ideological epiphenomena.

Genetic Risk and/as Governmentality

In many ways, the concept of governmentality has been developed and deployed as a way to avoid this kind of reduction. Often defined simply as the "conduct of conduct," the concept emerged for the first time in Foucault's Collège de France lectures in 1978 and 1979. In the February 1978 lecture titled "Governmentality," Foucault argued that as population overtook the family as the "plane of economy" in the early modern era, a new art of government began to form, one that stood in contrast to the sovereign power of the prince (100). As represented most infamously in Machiavelli's *The Prince*, the sovereign ruler stands in a singular and transcendent relationship to his principality; he and his rule are not part of the principality but rather they exercise dominion over it in order to increase their power. Thus, the end of sovereignty is circular, which is to say that the prince's aim is to keep and to strengthen his principality by exercising a juridical, warlike power (90, 95). The art of governing is, in contrast, plural and immanent, meaning that the state is governed according to a number of rational principles that emerge from it and cannot be derived from natural or divine law (97). Its objective is not one common good (the growth of the principality) but rather a number of ends that benefit those who are governed (95). Importantly, these goals are met not through the imposition of laws but rather through the "right disposition" of men and their relation to everything from wealth, resources, and the specific traits of the territory to customs, habits, accidents, and epidemics (93).

A common refrain in contemporary discussions of governmentality is that these ideas about modern government do not amount to a fully formed theory or point toward a clear method for studying all or any of the various ways in which we are governed. They were not robustly developed in Foucault's work, and most of the scholars who've come after Foucault insist that nothing like a school of thought has developed around them. These scholars often refer to governmentality as an "analytic," an "ethos of investigation," or a "way of asking questions" (Rose et al. 101). Yet for not constituting a coherent theory or school of thinking, governmentality has had a significant impact in the social sciences, where something of a "governmentality industry" has developed (Lemke 99). Scholars attribute this broad uptake, in part, to the way that governmentality illuminates "soft" or "empowering" forms of power in advanced neoliberal societies (Lemke 87). That is, in contrast to many strains of critical theory, especially Marxist, governmentality studies focus on how individuals produce the ends of government by fulfilling themselves rather than by simply obeying the law (Rose et al. 89). Several consequences follow from this orientation, with perhaps the most obvious being that the range of objects deemed suitable for analysis becomes much wider, expanding to include not just direct interventions by the state but also the "mundane practices and forms of subjectification" through which subjects create and conduct themselves as responsible, active citizens (Lemke 85).

However, this orientation also results in a kind of narrowing of purpose, insofar as it means that within governmentality studies there is no longer any recourse to freedom as a positive space for resistance to government (Rose et al. 91). Rather, freedom is understood as a key governmental strategy, one that replaces external regulation with internal production: subjects are produced as free so that they can be "responsibilized," which is to say, induced to identify dangers, calculate risks, and establish the necessary mechanisms of security to protect against them. This view of freedom, in turn, means that there is no place from within the analytic of governmentality to launch a critique of domination or to "look for the hidden in some deep structure" (Lemke 83). The aim, rather, is more modest if also more difficult: studies of governmentality "take programs at face value," analyzing how they identify and frame certain problems in order to make them amenable to "specific technical solutions" and produce "distinctive forms of expertise and moral problematization" (Lemke 83). Within such an effort, government cannot be approached as a "by-product" of social, economic, or cultural forces but instead is understood "as an attempt by those confronting certain social conditions to make sense of their environment, to imagine ways of improving the state of affairs, and to devise ways of achieving these ends" (Rose et al. 99). Nikolas Rose refers to this approach as an "agnosticism about 'why' and 'in whose interests' questions, accompanied by a commitment to studying how things get done" (93).

As Rose and others have pointed out, this kind of agnosticism does not, generally speaking, comport well with the goals ideology critique (Rose et al. 89; Lemke 80–83; Dean 35, 63–66). Yet if there is a topic around which the goals of governmentality studies and ideology critique have clearly merged, it is genetic risk. On the one hand, this merging is related to the lingering specter of eugenics. The destructive potential of genetic discrimination is so great, and the line between the "old" eugenics and the "new" genetics so subjective, that one imagines critics feel that they must remain on high alert for any development—a new scientific discovery, genetic test, or public health message—that, despite proclamations to the contrary, aims to distinguish the genetically fit from the unfit. On the other hand, however, it is also related to the fact that theories of risk associated with governmentality have taken strong constructivist positions on the nature of risk. Deborah Lupton, one of the most influential risk scholars in sociology, is very clear on this point, arguing that among social scientific theories of risk, "the govermentality perspective—taking its cue from Foucault's work on the discursive construction of reality—offers the most relativist position on risk" (*Risk and Sociocultural Theory* 6). She explains that those who work from this perspective are "not interested in investigating the nature of risk itself, but rather the forms of knowledge, the dominant discourses and expert techniques and institutions that serve to render risk calculable and knowable, bringing it into being" (6). What's significant about this constructivist understanding of risk isn't its epistemology per se but rather the kind of inquiry such an epistemology sets in motion. With the "nature of risk" and "forms of knowledge, dominant discourses, and expert techniques and institutions" so completely separated from one another, "how" questions are almost certain to slip into "why" questions. After all, if risk isn't real, then it only stands to reason that hidden forces have been at work "bringing it into being," and the critic's job is to identify those forces.

We can see this slippage from "how" to "why" questions most clearly, I would argue, by looking not to Foucault's work but rather to that of his Paris colleagues, François Ewald, a philosopher, and Robert Castel, a sociologist. Both Ewald and Castel published key essays on risk in the influential 1991 collection, *The Foucault Effect: Studies in Governmentality*. Ewald's essay addressed the function of risk within the context of insurance, arguing that whereas in everyday contexts risk typically refers to an objective threat or danger, its meaning within insurance is defined by three distinct traits: first, that it is calculable (202); second, that it is collective (203); and third, that it is capital, which is to say that what is insured isn't the injury or suffering itself but rather a value "against whose loss the insurer offers a guarantee" (204). More important than Ewald's delineation of these three traits, however (at least in terms of the essays' impact on future studies of risk), was his argument that insurers *produce* rather than find risks: "Nothing is a risk in itself," he wrote. "[T]here is no risk in reality. But on the other hand, anything *can* be a risk; it all depends on how one analyzes the danger, considers the event. As Kant might have put it, the category of risk is a category of the understanding; it cannot be given in sensibility or intuition" (199). Within the specific context of insurance, this view of risk points toward an obvious motive behind the construction of risks: financial gain. The more risks insurers manage to invent, the more profit they stand to make (199). But, taken out of the context of insurance, this view of risk points toward motive in general and that, in turn, puts the critic back in the familiar positions of decoder and debunker.

Castel's work on the function of risk within psychiatry provides a good example of this positioning. Broadly speaking, Castel was interested in how the movement within psychiatry from a preventative policy based on the classical notion of dangerousness to one based on the modern notion of risk facilitated the creation and circulation of what he called "the modern ideologies of prevention." Early preventive policy based on the notion of dangerousness was limited and crude because it located danger in a particular individual (283). Going beyond these methods meant breaking the direct connection to the individual, which is precisely what the modern notion of risk did (287). "A risk," Castel wrote, "does not arise from the presence of particular precise danger embodied in a concrete individual or group," but rather "is the effect of a combination of abstract *factors* which render more or less probable the occurrence of undesirable modes of behavior" (287). Thus, to know what counts as a risk, one does not start from an observable situation in experience but instead "*deduces* it from a general definition of the dangers one wishes to prevent" (287–88). Gone, then, is the "concrete subject of intervention," and in its place is a combination of "statistical correlations and heterogeneous elements" that are liable to produce risk (288). Within this paradigm, Castel contended, prevention assumes an ideological function, justifying the construction of a potentially unlimited number of new risks, as well as the idea that all risks should be eradicated, regardless of the iatrogenic effects such eradication might have (289).

While a number of the analyses of breast and ovarian cancer risk that I review below draw directly on Ewald or Castel, their influence has more often come through sociologists like Lupton, Alan Petersen, and Robin Bunton.[11] It is in their work that the merger between these two paradigms, ideology critique and governmentality studies, becomes most obvious. Take, for example, Lupton's very influential 1995 *The Imperative of Health: Public Health and the Regulated Body*. Here, Lupton turned to the concept of governmentality because she wanted to analyze the political implications of public health without simply condemning it for oppressing citizens' rights in order to benefit the state. Lupton rejected the view of power implicit in such a condemnation on the grounds that its dualisms (e.g., coercion versus consent) are too reductive to deal adequately with "the complexity of the nexus between public health, the state and other social institutions and apparatuses such as the family, the education system, mass media and commodity culture" (4). Governmentality provides a compelling alternative, she observed, because it views power relations as "diffuse, as emerging not necessarily from the state but from all areas of social life" (9). In light of this fact, Lupton argued that what matters about discourses of public health and health promotion are not the ways in which they "seek overtly to constrain individuals' freedom of action" but instead how they "invite individuals voluntarily to conform to their objectives, to discipline themselves, to turn the gaze upon themselves in the interest of their health" (11).

Lupton applied this analytic perspective in chapter 3, "Taming Uncertainty: Risk Discourse and Diagnostic Testing," using examples from discourses about HIV/AIDS, cholesterol, vaccines, prenatal care, breast cancer screening, and genetic testing, among other things, to demonstrate how risk operates as a political strategy in advanced neoliberal societies. Given the predominance of other theories of risk at the time (namely risk society theories), Lupton's ability to connect these and other discourses and practices of risk to the art of government is important. Yet the takeaway of these connections—the conclusion to which all of her analysis points—is that despite their objective, beneficent appearance, the fields of medicine and public health are just as politically motivated and ideological as recent critiques have shown science to be (104–5). More specifically, Lupton argued that while public health discourses of risk seem to be on the side of the public, the reality is that they use purportedly "objective medical and epidemiological classifications" to label particular individuals and groups as dangerous and assign then them moral blame and responsibility for poor health. This is obviously true in the case of internal or self-imposed risk since, for example, we can't easily blame the environment for eating too much. But Lupton argued that it's just as true in the case of external risk since locating ill health as a social rather than individual matter "simply shifts the blame from stigmatized individuals to the marginalized groups of which they are a member, while at the same time serving to obscure the suffering of individuals, who become anonymous 'risks' or 'threats' to the commonweal" (105). Thus, echoing Castel, she concluded that risk, as it is used in public health, "may be regarded as having less to do with the nature of 'danger' than the ideological purposes to which concerns about risk may be put" (105).

Alan Petersen's equally influential 1996 essay, "Risk and the Regulated Self: The Discourse of Health Promotion as a Politics of Uncertainty," followed a similar pattern. Troubled by the "metanarrative of progress and evolving self-consciousness" (46) underpinning the risk society theories, Petersen also turned to Castel, arguing that his understanding of risk is more suitable for critical analyses of public health because it not only draws attention to the power of experts to define and regulate subjects but also focuses on the new preventive strategies that characterize contemporary Western societies (47–48). Petersen connected these strategies to the political rationalities of neoliberalism, drawing on the work of scholars like Rose, Graham Burchell, and Colin Gordon to show in some detail how health promotion discourses encourage subjects to exercise a regulated autonomy, to live life as an enterprise, to enter into processes of their own self-governance and surveillance, and to pursue risk-free lives. But, again, the main point of drawing these connections was to show that despite the appearance of scientific rationality, health promotion is enmeshed in power relations and value judgments (56). Petersen called for more critical reflection on the values of entrepreneurialism, consumerism, and scientism that operate within the politics of health promotion, arguing that such reflection is necessary in order to extend citizen's rights and protect against covert forms of discrimination. "In a context of uncertainty," he warned, "all manner of interventions, what at other times or in other circumstances might be considered intrusive, oppressive, or discriminatory or paternalistic, can be justified as being for the protection of the 'at risk' individual and ultimately of benefit to society as a whole" (56). That there has not been enough reflection on these interventions and the values that undergird them stands as "testimony to the force of the modernist assumption that all problems can ultimately be controlled or eliminated through the pursuit of objective science and rational methods of control" (55).

Petersen extended this argument about the politics of health promotion to genetic risk two years later in his 1998 "The New Genetics and the Politics of Public Health," an essay in which, much like Duster, he warned that even though new genetic technologies could be beneficial, they were also capable of introducing "new and insidious forms of surveillance and control over 'problem populations'" (68). Genetic research is conducted "under the banner of 'disinterested science,'" he observed, "but it reinforces social divisions and "invariably conceal[s] conflicts of interest and relations of power" (69). Thus, again, Petersen called for critical analysis, asking, "[W]hat forms of surveillance, exclusion, and marginalization are associated with the new genetic screening and counseling services?" and "What, if any, scope is there for evading or resisting the more insidious forms of control implied by the 'geneticization' of health and disease?" (69).[12]

In studies like these, where the objective is to demonstrate that public health promotion is not as beneficent as it appears, governmentality becomes a way to avoid the perceived oversimplifications inherent in other forms of social and critical theory, but the concept does little to mitigate the hermeneutics of suspicion that stems from a constructivist view of risk. Thus, rather than illuminating qualitatively different *effects* of power, governmentality ends up pointing critics to different *channels* of power, namely to the practices individuals choose to participate in as a way to improve their health or reduce their health risks. But those choices are invariably revealed to be compulsory, and those practices, which are usually promoted by science, medicine, and public health as a form of empowerment, are invariably revealed to be a form of disempowerment. In governmentality-based studies of breast and ovarian cancer risk, this disempowerment is most often understood in terms of the heterosexist gender norms that operate in and through practices of cancer diagnosis and cancer prevention. Take, for example, Hallowell's 1999 "Doing the Right Thing: Genetic Risk and Responsibility" and Press et al.'s 2000 "Collective Fear, Individualized Risk: The Social and Cultural Context of Genetic Testing for Breast Cancer." Drawing on the work of scholars like Castel, Lupton, and Petersen, both studies sought to understand how risk works as a form of self-government within the specific context of genetic risk for breast and ovarian cancers. Hallowell's study, which was based on genetic counseling observations and patient interviews, found that even though genetic risk for breast and ovarian cancers is involuntary, it works as a form of self-government by engendering responsibility in much the same way that voluntary risk (e.g., smoking) does: by making disease prevention a moral issue. More specifically, however, her study found that this responsibility is the result of women's investment in "gendered discourses" that create an obligation not just to determine their risk and share it with family members (606–7) but also to manage their risk so that they can help others, for instance by being alive to raise their children (611) and by protecting family and friends from experiencing more cancer-related deaths (612). In light of these investments, Hallowell concluded that the responsibility felt by women at risk of breast and ovarian cancers diminished their autonomy, specifically their right not to know their genetic status (610) and not to undergo prevention practices that often have severe iatrogenic side effects (613). Importantly, Hallowell did note two exceptions to this conclusion—one, that because the women in her study actively sought genetic counseling, they could be seen as exercising autonomy; and two, that many interviewees rejected clinicians' advice and engaged in risk management practices even though they were determined to have a nonsignificant family pedigree (615). Yet rather than interpret these exceptions as evidence of actual autonomy, Hallowell interpreted them as evidence of the fact that women in the study had already invested in gendered discourses and been positioned as "at risk" before they came to the clinic (616).[13]

Press et al. came to a similar conclusion in their 2000 study, "Collective Fear, Individualized Risk," even though their object and method of analysis differed from Hallowell's. Rather than analyzing the discourses circulating through the narratives of at-risk women, they focused on the discourses embedded in—or "the forces that lie behind"—the diagnostics themselves, in this case, genetic susceptibility testing for BRCA1 and 2 mutations (247). Their main claim was that use of this technology depends on two related discourses: one, a discourse about breast cancer that teaches women to fear the disease, to overestimate their risk of developing it, and to believe in biomedicine's ability to cure it (240); and two, a discourse about risk that bases individual surveillance recommendations on population-level risk factors and promotes quantification (in the form of probability statistics) as a way to tame uncertainty (241–242). However, rather than actually quelling the cancer fears generated by the first discourse, they argued, this second discourse, the risk discourse, creates more fear by elaborating risk categories and defining those at risk as "not quite sick, but not quite well either" (242). "Anxiety about breast cancer is high," Press et al. wrote, "and a discourse of risk propels women endlessly forward in a quest for more information, while, in cyclical fashion, more information brings with it greater fear, anxiety, and hence *more* uncertainty and vigilant surveillance by women in the hope of protecting themselves from breast cancer" (247; emphasis added).

These breast cancer and risk discourses are not gendered in the same way that the ones under investigation in Hallowell's study are, but they do have gender-related effects insofar as the prevention practices toward which they channel women have the ability to "repress, control, and discipline women's bodies" (245). Specifically, Press et al. argued that recommendations to reduce risk by exercising, taking birth control, and having children young seem designed to "give women the bodies of boys or otherwise control their reproductive and sexual lives" and "undo the accomplishments women have achieved over the last 20 years" (245). The results of such efforts to "treat risk uncritically" are not only that other social values (e.g., women's autonomy) are ignored but also that risk becomes "a property of individual women" and thus an individual responsibility (246). This insight, in turn, points to what Press et al. identified as two key contradictions that characterize the use of these diagnostics: one, that while a technology like genetic susceptibility testing might be viewed by society in general as "liberating and potentially life-saving," others, for instance "a critical medical anthropologist," will observe it to be "repressive, punitive, and life-diminishing"; and two, that "individuals perceive themselves as free, liberated, and unconstrained while 'choosing' to use [such] a technology," but at the same time they have been "channeled towards that choice and normalized and disciplined through these same self-examinations" (239).

The last two studies I want to review here, Crabb and LeCouteur's "'Fiona Farewells Her Breasts': A Popular Magazine Account of Breast Cancer Prevention" and chapter 2 of Dubriwny's *The Vulnerable Empowered Woman*, "Genetic Risk: Prophylactic Mastectomy and the Pursuit of a Cancer-Free Life," also focus on processes of normalization and disciplining, but they do so by investigating a specific prevention practice, prophylactic bilateral mastectomy (PBM), rather than diagnostic practices. Given the date of these two studies, 2006 and 2013, respectively, this shift to prophylactic surgery makes sense. As genetic testing became more widespread after Myriad's BRC*Analysis* test was introduced in 1996, so did the use of PBM to manage risk. Not surprisingly, many critics wanted to understand how such a radical procedure could come to be perceived as an acceptable means of preventing a disease that even women with a diagnosed BRCA mutation were not certain to develop. From a constructivist perspective, the stakes in understanding this development are even higher since risk is taken to be a way of making sense of reality, not reality itself.[14] Thus, the question isn't just how does fear of breast cancer persuade women to remove healthy breasts but also what is happening rhetorically to make risk appear real.

Both Dubriwny and Crabb and LeCouteur answered these questions by analyzing what Dubriwny dubbed the "prophylactic mastectomy narrative," a cultural narrative that frames PBM as a "compulsory choice based on postfeminist expectations about femininity, sexuality, and reproduction" (Dubriwny 35). Both studies found that PBM is normalized and made "thinkable" within this narrative by two rhetorical patterns, one that positions women as mothers and another that equates genetic risk with cancer. The implications of this first pattern, positioning women as mothers, were borne out primarily through Crabb and LeCouteur's analysis of "'Fiona Farewells Her Breasts,'" a popular magazine article about an Australian woman who had a PBM to reduce her breast cancer risk. Crabb and LeCouteur argued that while this woman, Fiona, could have been identified in many ways, the article most consistently positioned her as a mother by explicitly referencing her children and by describing her relationship with them as central to her life and to her decision to have surgery (11). For instance, they noted that within the article a "discourse of motherhood as self-sacrifice" was used to justify the surgery as a way to prevent the suffering of Fiona's children when it could have been justified as a way to reduce her own suffering (12). Additionally, and echoing the findings of Hallowell's study, they observed that Fiona's desire to be alive to raise her children and to make sure they did not experience the loss of their mother was highlighted (12). Crabb and LeCouteur's point about these and other discursive constructions is that they made Fiona's decision seem "reasonable, correct, and morally responsible" (12). That is, by presenting Fiona, first and foremost, as a mother and by defining motherhood in terms of a willingness to engage in self-sacrifice, these constructions enable us to accept PBM as a rational choice (12). Within this textual pattern, then, the issue is ought: PBM is what a woman *ought* to do if she's a mother (13).

The second pattern of textual construction—equating genetic risk with cancer—is an issue of need, which is to say that PBM is presented as what women at risk *need* to do to stay alive (13). This depiction, in turn, depends on the construction of at-risk women as "patients without symptoms" (13). If we see them as people who are already not healthy and who are, in fact, destined to develop cancer, then PBM appears to be a perfectly rationale option. For instance, Crabb and LeCouteur argued that Fiona was never described as someone who was merely "at risk" of breast cancer, and, as a result, other prevention and surveillance options available to her were ignored (15). Dubriwny explained this same effect in terms of the narrative's organizational features, arguing that Jessica Queller's memoir of BRCA-related risk and prophylactic surgery, *Pretty Is What Changes*, obscured the difference between having risk and having cancer by beginning with a positive BRCA test result but then immediately moving back in time to reflect on Queller's mother's experience with cancer, which was agonizing for her and everyone who watched her die (52). According to Dubriwny, both this depiction of the cancer experience as agonizing and the decision to "ignore linear chronology" forged a close textual and emotional relationship between having genetic risk and having cancer (47). This relationship was reinforced by Queller's explanation of a post-PBM pathology report that revealed her to have atypical ductal hyperplasia in one breast. In Dubriwny's view, this pathology result, which Queller illustrated through a handful of similar anecdotes, left no space for being "simply 'BRCA positive'" (48–49). In other words, the message was that there's less difference between a bilateral mastectomy and a prophylactic bilateral mastectomy than we think because breast cancer is probably already developing (49). Thus, Dubriwny concluded, as did Crabb and

LeCouteur, that by collapsing risk and disease and by emphasizing the cancer experience of loved ones, the prophylactic mastectomy narrative is able to "situate cancer as an unacceptable risk and propel certain actions," namely making "the 'dramatic,' 'brave,' and 'radical' decision to have a prophylactic double mastectomy" (52). Yet the key point here—and, indeed, the conclusion reached in both Crabb and LeCouteur's and Dubriwny's analysis—is that this method of empowerment "is not a choice at all" (63). By framing breast cancer risk as unacceptable and by locating women's decisions within "a highly moralized context," the prophylactic mastectomy narrative not only leaves women with no space for questioning risk but also promotes a form of empowerment (surgical risk reduction) that, because it is justified by "traditional gendered configurations of home and family" must be acknowledged as a form of disempowerment (63).

Somewhere Other Than Critique

In my view, there is no question about the existence and the power of the prophylactic mastectomy narrative as Dubriwny has described it. Repeated over and over, this narrative seems almost ubiquitous now, showing up not just in mainstream media outlets and high-profile memoirs but also in the less public venues of support group websites, message boards, and personal blogs. In May of 2013, Angelina Jolie shocked the nation with her own version of the narrative, announcing, via a *New York Times* op-ed, that, after testing positive for a BRCA1 mutation, she had undergone a prophylactic bilateral mastectomy in order to reduce her risk of developing breast cancer. At the time of the op-ed, I remember thinking that for all the surprise Jolie's decision garnered among various sectors of the public, the way she framed that decision could not have been seen as anything other than completely predictable by critics in the humanities and social sciences. Indeed, Jolie's short—and tellingly titled—disclosure, "My Medical Choice," perfectly illustrates the traits of the prophylactic mastectomy narrative and the larger rhetoric of choice of which it is a part. Jolie told readers that once she knew of her mutation, she "decided to be proactive" and minimize her risk as much as possible by having surgery. While encouraging others with a family history of breast or ovarian cancers to "take action," Jolie was careful to highlight the importance of making one's "own informed choices." Yet, she justified her decision to have surgery through a rhetoric of maternal self-sacrifice, explaining that she was willing to do anything necessary to be with her children for as long as possible. Thus, while Jolie presented prophylactic surgery as her personal medical choice, from a constructivist perspective, we can clearly see how that choice was influenced by a history that says women's body parts (whether breasts or ovaries) are expendable, by an ideology that says science is objective, and by a set of heterosexist cultural discourses that says motherhood is a total commitment to and identification with one's children.

My aim in this chapter has been to demonstrate that the clarity with which we see these conclusions has, itself, become a problem. There's something counterintuitive about that statement, I realize. Arguably, clarity is a good thing, and the fact that we do, time and again, come to the same conclusions about the function of genetic risk suggests something about the correctness of those conclusions. But even if they are in some way correct, we have to ask if these conclusions are telling us anything new or allowing us to intervene in new ways. Because they consistently position us as decoders and debunkers, I worry that they aren't, that although they are satisfying to us, these conclusions are not doing for BRCA+ women what we want them to. Importantly, this worry does not stem from the kind of naïve realism that says we should simply accept genetic medicine's claims of better health through personal choice. Nor does it stem from the idea that if those at risk feel empowered by their decisions to be "proactive," as Jolie put it, then they are, in fact, empowered. It stems, rather, from the belief that, like the patients described in Mol's *The Logic of Care*, those at genetic risk of disease experience a lack of freedom that cannot be remedied by enlightenment or emancipation. This belief, in turn, leads me to the conclusion, or at least to the hypothesis, that much of what they say and do escapes the questions of choice and empowerment that have dominated the arguments of both genetic medicine and its critics for more than two decades now. Thus, we have to aim for something other than critique. As Latour reminds us, this does not mean that we have to stop being critical. It means, rather, that we need to cultivate new ways of being critical. Despite over two decades of thoroughgoing critique, there are no signs that the use of presymptomatic genetic testing is abating. Despite legitimate concerns about genetic medicine's potential to exacerbate political and social inequities, to lead to genetic discrimination and determinism, and to normalize extreme medical interventions through rhetorics of disease prevention, thousands of people find the arguments of the new genetics persuasive enough to act on them, that is, to undergo presymptomatic genetic testing and to engage in surveillance and prevention practices. My wager here is that we can learn something new about the experience of being at genetic risk—and we can respond to rhetorics of choice more effectively—if our critical efforts don't begin with the assumption that this persuasion is primarily the result of ideological manipulation. However, if we are to do that, that is, if we are to end up somewhere other than critique, then we have to begin somewhere other than constructivism.

3

Making Risk Real | A Praxiographic Inquiry into Being BRCA+

Most of us are probably familiar with Kaplan's law of the instrument, even if we don't recognize it by that name. It's the simple adage that if all you have is a hammer, then everything you see will look like a nail. In essence, this is the point I tried to demonstrate in chapter 2—that as long as we are operating with a constructivist understanding of genetic risk, then we are almost certainly going to end up engaged in critique, and it makes little difference if that understanding is deployed within the theoretical apparatus of ideology or within the theoretical apparatus of governmentality. The results are the same: beginning with the idea that risk is not real, we try to identify the discursive mechanisms by which it has been made to seem real. We show, for instance, how women who have risk-reducing surgeries believe they are making free choices when in fact they are making compulsory choices; we show how rhetorical constructions of at-risk women promote forms of empowerment that are actually disempowering because they reinforce heterosexist gender norms; and we show that for all of its talk of epigenetics and environmental influence, the new genetics is just as deterministic as its predecessor, eugenics. In short, we operate as debunker, distinguishing appearance from reality in the hopes that women at genetic risk will be able to make better, which is to say (somewhat ironically) freer, choices. In this sense, we might say that constructivist critiques don't dislodge the rhetoric of choice surrounding genetic risk as much as they provide another version of it.

If we don't want to end up in the role of debunker, then where do we begin? What kind of understanding of BRCA risk do we need? We need to understand BRCA risk as something that is real, but, as I argued in chapter 2, we can't slide back into the kind of naïve realism that would enact the same kind of purification, only in the opposite direction.[1] Such a move would again separate nature from culture, leaving us this time with an understanding of BRCA risk as a simple matter of fact: the result of an altered, deleted, or added nucleotide in a gene on chromosome 17 or 13. In *Reassembling the Social*, Latour refers to this move as social constructivism's "symmetric error" because it assumes that nature is the mute stuff of interpretation, that is, the stable reality on which we can take multiple perspectives. In this way of thinking, multiplicity exists only on the side of the social, while nature, which is granted some degree of "realness," is thought to be unified and indisputable or, in other words, nonsocial. But for Latour, neither this division nor the theory of "interpretive flexibility" it promotes can describe the "highly uncertain and loudly disputed [. . .] real, objective, atypical and, above all, *interesting* agencies" that populate our world (114). For that task, a new category must be introduced: *matters of concern*. Borrowing from Heidegger, Latour defines matters of concern as *gatherings*, that is, as objects capable of bringing together the elements of the fourfold—earth, sky, gods, and mortals ("Why Has Critique Run Out of Steam?" 235). But while Heidegger reserved this term, "gatherings," only for the "thingness" of Things, those artifacts "cradled in the respectful idiom of arts, craftsmanship, and poetry," Latour applies it more broadly, arguing that industrially made objects, including those of science and technology, should be acknowledged as having the "rich and complicated qualities" of the Thing (233–34). In his view, such an acknowledgment would go a long way in promoting a kind of critical engagement that seeks to get close to the objects of science and technology in order to care for them, not debunk them.

By disentangling the quality of being real from the qualities of being unified and indisputable (or nonsocial), Latour's notion of matters of concern provides a first and, I think, essential step toward figuring out how to grant BRCA risk some reality without moving back to a place of naïve realism. Moreover, it reminds us that we can try to get close to BRCA risk in order to explain it without the goal of critiquing or debunking it. Yet it does not tell us *how* to get close to that object. Latour's own work with actor-network theory (ANT) points to one possibility, and there is no doubt that a description of the network of human and nonhuman actants that has enabled BRCA risk to emerge as an object would help us get close to it. But as John Law argues, ANT-inspired studies have tended to privilege science and technology as the key sites of reality production and thus inscription devices as the key means of reality production ("Enacting Naturecultures" 6). This focus has been "unduly restricting," he maintains, insofar as it has turned attention away from public understandings of science, focusing it on the "more or less coherent, more or less stabilized, rather obdurate" realities emerging from laboratories (5). In order to broaden our view to include questions about public understandings of science (but using ontological rather than epistemological terms[2]), Law points to what he calls "the third great version of STS," the "turn to enactment," which posits that all sorts of practices beyond the lab participate in the making, unmaking, and remaking of realties, and that they often do so in order to intervene—to "make a difference in a body or a life"—rather than to describe or tell (5–7).

This turn to enactment is nowhere better illustrated and explained than in *The Body Multiple: Ontology in Medical Practice*, Annemarie Mol's 2002 praxiographic study of the artery disease atherosclerosis. In brief, praxiography is like ethnography insofar as the goal is to understand some phenomenon from an insider's perspective. But whereas in most ethnographies that phenomenon is typically some aspect of culture, in praxiography, the object under investigation is practice or, more specifically, how practices bring objects into being by enacting them in various ways. In *The Body Multiple*, Mol follows atherosclerosis around a hospital in the Netherlands, observing procedures, sitting through consultations, and listening to what patients say about living with impaired bodies and to what physicians say about treating them. She finds that because atherosclerosis is enacted through multiple practices across many sites, it has multiple realities, and her goal is to explain how these various realities are coordinated through processes like addition and calibration. The multiplicity that necessitates this coordination does not make atherosclerosis less real; but it does mean that its "realness" cannot be understood as coming from a unified, indisputable foundation, for example, nature. If an object like atherosclerosis is real, Mol argues, then "this is because it is part of a practice. It is a reality enacted" (44).

BRCA risk is not an object like atherosclerosis, which is to say that it is not a disease with its own symptoms, treatments, specialists, and clinics. Highly distributed and poorly defined, BRCA risk is what John Law and Vicky Singleton would call a "messy object." Messy objects cannot be "narrated smoothly" from a single location (348), and they have such porous borders that the researchers who study them (and the people who deal with them) often find their focus slipping onto other objects (Law, *After Method* 79). But messy objects are enacted in practices every day, and, by Mol's logic, these enactments—as multiple and incongruous as they might be—make them real. BRCA risk is no exception to this logic and, in fact, could be seen as a paradigmatic example of it. Every day, thousands of women enact BRCA risk through practices that compress, palpate, and image their bodies, that alter their anatomies and biochemistries, that change what they eat and drink, that affect how (or if) they have sex, if they sleep well at night, if they breastfeed their children, and how they dress. We could even argue that outside of these practices, BRCA risk has no reality of its own, meaning that either it does nothing (i.e., has no discernible effect on health) or fades to the background as a different but related object—cancer—comes on the scene. Thus, no matter what meaning we attach to BRCA risk, no matter how we've explained its conditions of possibility, it needs to be understood as something that women *do* and as something whose realities, therefore, are not just scientific or ideological.

My goal in this chapter, then, is to use praxiography as a way to get close to the enacted realities of BRCA risk, to treat it as a matter of concern, in other words. But because executing a full praxiographic study of this messy object would be the job of an entire book, not one chapter in a book, I have narrowed my approach here by focusing on one kind of practice associated with BRCA risk—breast cancer screening. Anyone with even a passing familiarity of the "BRCA experience" will recognize cancer screening as one of the two choices that BRCA+ women can make once they've learned of their mutation status. Through practices like mammography and breast MRI, they can try to catch breast cancer early, when it's more treatable. Or, through practices like bilateral mastectomy and/or chemoprevention, they can try to reduce their chances of developing cancer.[3] Historically speaking, we have tended to pay more attention to this latter set of practices, and to some degree, that disparity is understandable. Cancer screening is more familiar to us; certain forms of it (e.g., mammography and colonoscopy) eventually become part of many people's regular health-care regimen. And, more important, cancer screening is not perceived to be a drastic response to BRCA risk. It doesn't put women through major surgeries (and the severe iatrogenic side effects that can accompany them) in order to prevent cancer by removing healthy organs. It allows them to be "simply 'BRCA positive,'" as Dubriwny puts it (50).

But this doesn't mean that breast cancer-screening practices don't do anything. More than one option in a choice that no one wants to make, breast cancer screening is a way that BRCA risk comes to have a reality in the lives of women at genetic risk of breast and ovarian cancers. Drawing on interviews with BRCA+ women, as well as a variety of the medical and biosocial discourses that surround BRCA risk, I try to show that this reality is one that often overlaps with the reality of disease. As we know from chapter 2, this is not a particularly novel claim to make. Using a rhetorical methodology, Happe showed us how risk and disease overlap in ways that make PBSO "thinkable" for BRCA+ women, while Crabb and LeCouteur and Dubriwny did the same for PBM, arguing that rhetorical patterns in the "PM narrative" equate risk with cancer, thus framing the surgery as something BRCA+ women need to do. Though I do not doubt that risk and disease overlap in the ways that they describe, my claim here is different insofar as the overlap I wish to highlight is one that we cannot debunk, one that will not go away, in other words, once our rhetorical analyses have brought it to light. Importantly, this does not mean that the reality of BRCA risk and the at-risk body that I seek to describe is *the* reality, unchangeable and unified. Even if I am focusing on just one type of practice in this chapter, the key insight of praxiography is that reality is multiple because practices are multiple. So while I do want to show that breast cancer-screening practices enact BRCA risk and the at-risk body in such a way that risk and disease really do—that is, *in reality*—overlap, I do not want to suggest that this is the way things will always be. Indeed, I hope that as screening practices change, so will the realities of BRCA risk and the at-risk body. At this time, though, when genetic medicine is "technologically ahead of the curve and diagnostically behind [it]," as one BRCA+ woman put it (Falls), there is overlap, and that overlap, I will argue here, can be seen in the way that breast cancer screening enacts BRCA risk as a chronic condition, that is, something that can be managed and monitored through tests but that can never go away and will, in fact, "get worse" (i.e., increase) over time. Further, I will try to show that through those tests, the at-risk body is turned into a source of knowledge about cancer. Turning the at-risk body into a source of knowledge about cancer is not the same thing as having cancer, but it does create opportunities for risk and disease to overlap, particularly through the problem of false positive test results on breast MRI. I explain this problem in some detail in the second half of the chapter, ultimately arguing that it is precisely the kind of constraint in medicine that necessitates a rhetoric of care. Before I make that argument, though, I want to briefly review praxiography and explain my use of it in this chapter.

Reviewing Praxiography

As I've explained, Mol defines praxiography as the study of how objects come into being by virtue of their enactment in practice. In her work, the objects under investigation are usually medical objects, and the aim is to explain how procedures, technologies, and instruments enact or "do" them. Methodologically speaking, this means that researchers must not only focus on practices but also that they must operate in "a realist mode," an imperative that, until recently, would have been anathema in many corners of rhetorical studies (*Body Multiple* 15). What Mol means by "realist" here is arguably very similar to Jane Bennett's call for moments of "methodological naiveté" or "a suspension of genealogical critique" in order to "render manifest a subsistent world of nonhuman vitality" (17). Mol doesn't talk in terms of "nonhuman vitality" or work out of the Spinozian/Deluezian philosophical tradition that influences Bennett, but she is very much interested in the agency of things, particularly illnesses and the material objects—tables, microscopes, scalpels, catheters, and so on—that enact them. In addition, Mol believes that operating in a "realist mode" means listening to people who are ill as though they can act as their own ethnographers, as though they are the insiders when it comes to disease. But, in contrast to a more traditional ethnographic approach, this listening is not focused on those elements of experience that we accept as inevitably subjective, such as perspectives, feelings, and meanings. Rather the researcher here listens in order to understand how "living with an impaired body is *done* in practice" (*Body Multiple* 15; emphasis added). Through this kind of listening, Mol argues, an illness emerges that is "both material and active," that consists of countless material and practical realities, and that the patient both does and has done to them (20).

Thinking of illness as something that patients do and have done to them stands in contrast to two more common moves in the social sciences—the first, to conceive of illness as an important psychosocial counterpart to the physicalities of disease, which are the physician's province; and the second, to argue that whatever physicians say about the disease is a result of their perspective as biomedical insiders (12–13). Combined, Mol argues, these moves have created a narrow area of inquiry within medicine for the social sciences, one where "physical reality fades from view" and researchers are left to interpret the various meanings of illness. Within this tradition, different interpretations abound, but "the disease—forever unknown—is nowhere to be found" (11–12). Praxiography counters this tradition by providing a way for social scientists (and humanists) to study the sick body not only as it is interpreted by the patient or the doctor, but also as it is practically performed or enacted, that is, as it is "manipulated, measured, observed, cut into pieces—or grows and decays" ("Missing Links, Making Links" 162). Thus, physical reality is reclaimed, but, echoing Latour, Mol emphasizes that it is not reclaimed as a unified, indisputable foundation: "The aim is to breach the dividing line between human subjects and natural objects—but not in a way such that physics can take over the world, or that genetics is allowed to explain us all. The (serious) game played here makes a move that is the other way around: like (human) subjects, (natural) objects are framed as part of events that occur and plays that are staged. If an object is real this is because it is part of a practice. It is a reality *enacted*" (*Body Multiple* 44).

As Mol repeatedly points out, the logic here is simple, but its implications are far reaching: if reality is the result of practices, and practices are multiple, then reality is also multiple. This is the primary lesson of *The Body Multiple*, which, as I noted earlier, is a study of how the common artery disease, atherosclerosis, is enacted across different sites in a Dutch hospital. The version of atherosclerosis that is enacted in the hospital's outpatient clinic, for instance, is incompatible with the version that is enacted in its pathology lab; in Mol's terms, they *exclude* one another insofar as the first requires a patient who complains about pain in his legs, while the second requires a cross section of an artery visible under the microscope (35). Mol stresses that this incompatibility is not an issue of failed translation or of the conflicting perspectives of surgeons and pathologists, professionals whom she has observed as quite capable of talking to and understanding one another. The incompatibility, rather, is a practical matter of how atherosclerosis is done differently in different sites (36).

Adapting Praxiography

Mol's work has been well received and widely applied across the humanities and social sciences in large part because of the rapprochement with reality it offers. Praxiography allows researchers to talk about what an object *is*, how it exists physically in the world, but the meaning of "is" has changed. The new "is" is situated and multiple, never saying what something is in and of itself and never bracketing the practicalities that are involved in enacting reality (54). Moreover, by making this move toward an understanding of reality as multiple, praxiography has provided a much-needed alternative to perspectivalism and constructivism, both of which theorize reality as plural. In the case of perspectivalism, to say that reality is plural is to say that because people come from different backgrounds, they will inevitably see objects in different ways. Yet the object itself sits in the middle of these perspectives, "singular, untouched, intangible" (Mol, "Ontological Politics" 76). Constructivism, on the other hand, tells us that reality is plural because it can be constructed in any number of ways, but the version that we accept as true is the one that has emerged, victorious, intact, and more or less coherent, over its competitors. Neither theory, Mol argues, gives reality a "complex present," which is to say that neither allows us to acknowledge that different versions of an object can exist simultaneously, and that these versions are either sustained or allowed to fade away depending on the demands of local circumstances.

Mol's emphasis not just on location but on "localness" marks another reason for praxiography's appeal, namely its approach to politics. Praxiography is, in some sense, all about surfaces. The aim, as Mol says many times, is to go inside medicine, but it's to go inside in order to look *at* the practices that enact diseases and bodies, not *behind* them for hidden forces or agendas. In other words, the focus is on describing and assessing the local value of various enactments of diseases and bodies, not on interpreting their meaning within a larger social or ideological system (Mol, "Missing Links, Making Links" 163). Arguably, there is no area of biomedicine where such a focus is needed more than in genetic medicine, where polarizing arguments about hidden eugenic agendas and the promises of personalized medicine have obscured how genetic risk is enacted in medical practice and in the daily lives of those at risk. Praxiography opens up these practices, allowing us to do something other than take a stand "for" or "against" genetic medicine, an important move in its own right but also one that is necessary for developing the rhetoric of care that is the subject of chapter 4.

For all of this appeal, though, executing a praxiographic study is not a straightforward matter of replicating Mol's method in a different context. Because praxiographies are so site- and object-specific, researchers must tailor their methods to the material studied, a process that often begins by identifying what Christian Bueger refers to as alternative "empirical access points" (1). In *The Body Multiple*, the empirical access point is a physical site, a hospital in the Netherlands that hosts "a dense ensemble of practices" (Bueger 10). And while Mol employs many data collection strategies within that site (e.g., archival work, interview, and document analysis), she relies chiefly on participant observation, visiting the hospital once or twice a week to sit through consultations, to watch technicians work in labs, to witness operations, and to attend meetings where difficult cases are discussed (Mol, *Body Multiple* 1–3). Mol's access to practices inside the hospital was not unlimited, but it was certainly extensive and, in many ways, ideal; having gone to medical school herself, Mol was seen as an insider by many of the doctors in the hospital. But most researchers don't have this kind of access, and often logistics, resources, and the "intricacies of observation" necessitate reliance on alternative access points and data collection strategies (Bueger 17). Controversy, for instance, can be an entry point into a praxiographic study when access to a physical site isn't possible or appropriate. The idea here, according to Bueger, is that when actors are at odds about the practices they participate in—a situation that often arises when a new practice is introduced or existing ones appear incompatible—they become more reflexive about how those practices work, as well as the values and rationales embedded in them. This reflexiveness, then, becomes an opportunity for initiating a praxiographic study. Scott Graham and Carl Herndl's 2013 study of pain treatment controversy, "Multiple Ontologies in Pain Management: Toward a Post-plural Rhetoric of Science," illustrates this type of praxiography. By conducting expert interviews, attending professional meetings, and analyzing a variety of documents (e.g., mission statements, scholarly articles, and textbooks), Graham and Herndl examined how members of the Midwest Pain Group (MPG) interacted with one another despite having vastly different approaches to pain treatment, for example, administering cognitive-behavioral therapy versus administering opiate pharmaceuticals. What they found is that "nested" within the particular practices of the clinicians were six different pain ontologies, that is, six different ways of enacting the nature of pain, and that these ontologies, not conflicting conceptual schemes or paradigms, were responsible for the discursive differences that characterized the group (117, 122). Graham substantially extended this work in his 2015 *The Politics of Pain Medicine: A Rhetorical-Ontological Inquiry*, a book that explains how the MPG functions as a "metapractical site" where various presentational genres and deliberative practices achieve the work of "ontological calibration," thus allowing for the ongoing development of nonmodern pain ontologies that reject the Cartesian mind/body divide (88, 65). Graham terms his study of these rhetorical processes of calibration a "praxiography of representation" and offers it as a way of bringing rhetoric and STS together for the sake of a "robust rhetorical-ontological account of pain science and medicine" (22).

For others, entry into a praxiographic study comes from following an artifact across time or space in order to investigate the practices through which it emerged, as well as those that are "inscribed" within it (Bueger 16). Bueger refers to this approach as an "object ethnography," and while that phrase is broad enough to describe any type of praxiography, he uses it to draw attention to the fact that praxiographic studies can begin not only with physical artifacts but also with "conceptual" ones, that is, with artifacts that result from, assemble, and enable certain types of practices but are not tangible things like water pumps or blood sugar monitors (16). Diedrich and Boyce's 2007 "Breast Cancer on Long Island: The Emergence of a New Object Through Mapping Practices" is a good example of this type of object ethnography. Interested in how different mapping practices produced different versions of a specific medical object, "breast cancer on Long Island," Diedrich and Boyle examined three cases, a ten-foot pin map of incidences of breast cancer created by local activists, a space-cluster analysis published by two geographers, and a zip code–based report from the New York Cancer Surveillance Improvement Initiative. After explaining how the activists' pin map brought "breast cancer on Long Island" into existence, they show how the two subsequent maps worked to unmake that existence by portraying activists as nonexperts whose methods could not lead to scientific knowledge and by stressing the link between cancer and lifestyle rather than cancer and the environment (207).

Geertje Mak's 2012 *Doubting Sex: Inscriptions, Bodies, and Selves in Nineteenth-Century Hermaphrodite Case Histories* is also an object ethnography that moves back in time to demonstrate how an object came into existence, but in this case that object—hermaphroditism—is understood as an act, specifically, the act of doubting sex. Mak's central question is how did different nineteenth-century medical practices establish the ability to doubt biological sex? How did one know, for instance, that a body could or could not ejaculate sperm? By palpating a patient's genitals? By looking at sperm in a microscope? By examining stains on a bedsheet? Mak's argument is that the practices through which such facts were established operated according to tacit logics and produced sex in historically and geographically distinct ways (8). What's important about this argument (besides its findings, which are too numerous to summarize here) are its materials and Mak's method of analyzing them. Because her work is historical, Mak had to rely solely on texts (medical case histories and autobiographies) for evidence about practices. Thus, veering from the kind of critical or symptomatic reading more common in the humanities, she chose to read those texts referentially, accepting that if a practice was described in a certain way, it happened in that way. If a physician said that he "carefully palpated a testicle, epididymis and spermatic cord," for example, then Mak took him at his word, reading in a realist mode and treating him as his own ethnographer (8).

A Praxiographic Inquiry into Being BRCA+

The praxiographic study of BRCA risk that I present here does not perfectly mirror any of those reviewed above, including and, perhaps especially, Mol's, where the object of study is about as uncontroversial as a medical object can be. Yes, doctors and patients disagree about the nature and treatment of atherosclerosis, but it is not a disease that we think of as politicized. Not so in the case of BRCA risk. While it is a medical object, it is not a disease, and for that reason alone it is highly politicized. But add to that the politics of cancer culture (and, in particular breast cancer culture) and the result is a medical object that could not be more different from the mundane artery disease at the center of Mol's study. Thus, as I argued in chapter 1, there's a great deal at stake in trying to demonstrate that BRCA risk is real rather than a social construction. Moreover, the fact that this is my primary goal here—to demonstrate that BRCA risk is, praxiographically speaking, real—marks another key difference between my study and Mol's. Mol demonstrated not just that atherosclerosis is real but that it has multiple realities depending on how it is enacted in various practices. While I hope that my study implies the same about BRCA risk (that if we studied a different set of practices, we would see it enacted as a different kind of object), I have not made its multiple realities my focus here. In large part, this is an issue of space—the fact that, as I said earlier, it would take an entire book to execute a full praxiographic study of this messy object. But it's also an issue of purpose: if my aim here is to show, against a long-standing constructivist tradition, that it is possible to talk about BRCA risk as something that is real, then going into detail about one mode of enactment seemed a better bet than providing a more cursory investigation of two or three modes of enactment.

Two additional differences between my study and Mol's warrant mentioning: one, the fact that care for BRCA+ women is so decentralized, spread over the offices of many types of physicians—oncologists, plastic surgeons, gynecologists, and radiologists, for instance—that it cannot easily be followed through one physical site in the way that atherosclerosis can be; and two, the fact that even if it could be followed through one physical site, my professional training as a rhetorician does not provide the same level of access as Mol's medical school background. Like the other scholars whose work I've reviewed here, then, I have relied on alternative data sources and data collection strategies to follow an object across the discourses of relevant stakeholders in order to understand how it is enacted by a specific set of practices. Not surprisingly, the discourses I have relied on most heavily are those produced by BRCA+ women. Over the course of four months in the end of 2014 and the beginning of 2015, I conducted ten in-depth interviews with BRCA+ women, asking them mainly open-ended questions but also encouraging them to tell me, in the most specific and practical terms possible, what living with a BRCA mutation is like.[4] In addition and over a much longer period of time, I read a variety of biosocial BRCA-related texts, including but not limited to op-eds, BRCA guidebooks, memoirs, and ninety-one threads (totaling 137 pages of text) from the main forum of the FORCE message boards.[5] My reading of all of this discourse was guided by two broad research questions: One, what is BRCA risk when enacted through cancer-screening practices; and two, how do those practices enact or do the at-risk body? Coming up with answers to these questions was essentially a matter of reading referentially in the way Mak describes; that is, I listened to what BRCA+ women said they did and what they said they had done to them and assumed, as Mol did in *The Body Multiple*, that they were the insiders when it came to living with BRCA risk. In addition, I focused as much as possible on the practicalities, material objects, technologies, and techniques that appeared in their stories, believing that this was the best way to "follow" BRCA risk and allow it to take shape as something that is "both material and active" (Mol, *Body Multiple* 20).

Reading referentially in this way led me to two observations: one, that when enacted in the mode of cancer screening, BRCA risk becomes a kind of chronic condition, that is, something that can be managed and monitored through tests but never "cured"; and two, that these tests enact or do the at-risk body as a source of knowledge about cancer. From these observations, I reached the broader conclusion that in this mode of enactment, the reality of BRCA risk is one that overlaps with the reality of disease. While the discourses of BRCA+ women helped me come to this conclusion, they were not sufficient for explaining it, at least not in any technical way. Thus, I turned to the discourses of another kind of stakeholder—the researchers, clinicians, and technicians who study and/or conduct breast cancer screening for high-risk women. I did this in a number of ways, first by attending the June 2015 FORCE annual conference, "Joining Forces Against Hereditary Cancer," where I heard panels on topics ranging from breast cancer surveillance and menopause management to targeted cancer therapies and communicating genetic information. Also at this conference I was able to go to "ask the expert" sessions where conference attendees could sit and talk with clinicians across a range of specializations in an informal setting. Then, as my argument began to focus more specifically on the problem of false positive test results for breast MRI, I started reading research articles and medical textbook chapters about high-risk breast cancer–screening protocols, procedures, and controversies. I also read or watched a good deal of patient-facing material about high-risk breast cancer screening, including, for instance, hospital website pages and instructional videos about MRI-guided breast biopsy. Through this reading and watching, I again tried to follow BRCA risk, but this time through a fairly technical set of discourses about a specific set of radiologic screening and diagnostic practices. Lack of medical training posed some challenges for understanding this material, and so in July of 2016, I set up an interview with Dr. Barrett, a diagnostic radiologist at a nearby breast-imaging center. Although my primary reason for interviewing Dr. Barrett was to gain a better understanding of some of the more technical aspects of the procedures I had been reading about, it became clear during our conversation that he was also an important ethnographer of the events through which BRCA risk is enacted. A longer, more sustained praxiographic study of BRCA risk would surely benefit from including more interviews with clinicians like Dr. Barrett who do BRCA risk.

The Logistical Messiness of BRCA Risk

Doing BRCA risk through cancer-screening practices is often referred to as "watchful waiting" in BRCA guidebooks, and while the "watchful" part of that phrase certainly captures the vigilance that screening requires, the "waiting" part implies a kind of passivity that is not borne out in first-person accounts of living with BRCA risk. BRCA+ women who manage their risk through screening *do* a lot. The current National Comprehensive Cancer Network's (NCCN) standard of care surveillance guidelines for women at high risk[6] of breast and ovarian cancers include:

+ Breast awareness beginning at age twenty-five[7]
+ Clinical breast exams every six to twelve months beginning at age twenty-five
+ Alternating mammograms and breast MRIs every six months beginning at age twenty-five or five to ten years before the earliest case of breast cancer in the family

+ Pelvic exam, transvaginal ultrasound, and CA-125 testing every six to twelve months starting at age thirty or five to ten years before the earliest case of ovarian cancer in the family.[8]

Together, these screening practices create a regimen of doctor's appointments that has no natural endpoint. Thus, as I explained at the outset, one key claim of my argument here is that screening enacts BRCA risk as a chronic condition insofar as it never goes away. Risk cannot be "cured," and, in fact, increases over time as a woman ages. In the case of breast cancer, risk can also increase when an abnormality is detected through screening or biopsy, even if that abnormality is determined to be benign. When enacted in this mode, then, BRCA risk cannot be reduced, but it can be managed and monitored by tests that check a whole host of features, for instance, antigen levels, densities, growths, thicknesses, contours, enhancement patterns, calcification clusters, cellular structures, and so on. These tests are obviously performed on bodies, and so another key claim in my argument is that within the mode of screening, the body is made to be a source of knowledge. It has to be read, interpreted, and figured out in order to manage and monitor BRCA risk.[9]

But that's not really the case, is it? The body is not turned into a source of knowledge about risk—it's turned into a source of knowledge about cancer. All of the screening practices that BRCA+ women participate in make the body readable in order to know if its cells have begun proliferating uncontrollably and produced a malignancy. Here, in this slippage from risk to cancer, we can see why it's fitting to think of BRCA risk as a messy object: its border with cancer is very porous, and, as a result, these two objects often overlap with one another. While I will eventually explain this overlap between risk and disease in terms of specific cancer-screening practices, I want to begin more generally, as many accounts of BRCA risk do, with some of the practicalities that characterize a typical cancer-screening routine, for instance, where it takes place, how often it takes place, and who performs it. Although a number of major medical centers offer comprehensive, centralized screening programs for high-risk patients (Memorial Sloan Kettering's RISE program is a good example), most BRCA+ women must coordinate their own screening regimen. Hannah, a thirty-three-year-old BRCA2+ college professor explained that this is how "being BRCA+" began for her, by "trying to figure out who is supposed to care for you and where you go and when you go to them." Like most of the women I interviewed, Hannah didn't know who was supposed to care for her. Efforts to make appointments with specialists were met with requests for referrals and admonitions that she couldn't "just schedule" her own appointments. Eventually, with the help of a medical social worker, Hannah got an appointment to see the "big shot" oncologist in her town, but, in her case, access didn't translate into understanding or medical care. When she requested ovarian cancer screening she was told there was no way she could have ovarian cancer at her age and was given a referral to a psychiatrist. Nancy, a BRCA2+ fifty-six-year-old technical writer, explained a similar experience, noting how "weird" it was when the oncologist she visited began their consultation by asking how she felt about her body. "I didn't quite get that, unless that was her way of wanting to know if I was considering mastectomy. I don't know, but let's just say we didn't click. She was like, 'Why are you here? You don't have cancer.' Then I wondered why my doctor sent me to her, too."

The point here isn't that these doctors were bad oncologists, though it is hard to ignore the paternalism of an unsolicited psych referral. The point, rather, is that Hannah and Nancy didn't have cancer and yet they needed to be under the care of doctors who specialize in treating cancer. This is a practical issue, one that not only produces scheduling difficulties and awkward exchanges but also means spending time in cancer care centers or oncology offices, places where the physical realities of disease are unavoidable. For many BRCA+ women, visiting the oncologist means seeing the future they fear most. That sounds crass and unfair to cancer patients, but it's true, as Carrie, a thirty-six-year-old BRCA1 mutation carrier, explained. She felt this fear about the future most acutely when sitting in the waiting room at the cancer center office of her gynecologic oncologist. "I sat there in the waiting room full of women with headscarves and IV drips, and my blood pressure went through the roof. When I looked around, I said to my husband, 'That's not going to be me. I'm not doing that.' I love my gynecologist but I told her, 'I'm not going to come back to you anymore, because I can't keep coming to your hospital.'" Hannah also emphasized physical location when I asked if she ever found an oncologist to perform ovarian cancer screening. She had, but it was a two-part process that typically took a couple of hours at the cancer center. First, to get the transvaginal ultrasound, she went down to the cancer center's radiology department, where "this dildo thing" scanned her ovaries. Then, for the second part of the appointment, she met with the oncologist, who "performed the physical exam, a pelvic exam, a blood test, all of that stuff." But in between was a couple of hours spent in a waiting room "full of people with cancer, mostly women, bald women, women holding catheter bags full of urine, women with oxygen tanks, women who are clearly dying of ovarian cancer or breast cancer or who are going through chemo." "I am usually the only healthy-looking one there," Hannah explained, "so it's really bizarre and stressful."

What can make this experience even more stressful for BRCA+ women is the number of times it must be repeated. How the NCCN surveillance guidelines are actually put into practice varies across individual patients, doctors, and institutions, but most of the women I interviewed and whose accounts I read described going to four to seven appointments a year, and that was not counting follow-up scans or biopsies. For Lizzy Stark, author of the popular BRCA memoir, *Pandora's DNA*, the NCCN guidelines meant seven appointments a year, which was enough to leave her feeling like she had been "felt up and fingered by every clinician in the state" (120). Part of the problem in her case was logistical. While the NCCN recommendation of one mammogram and one MRI per year might sound like two doctor's appointments, for Stark it was four since each scan required a preliminary visit to the oncologist who performed a clinical breast exam and ordered the imaging tests (121). In *Blood Matters*, another popular BRCA memoir, journalist Masha Gessen describes participating in a screening regimen similar to Stark's, but for her an annual breast MRI was actually two separate procedures, "owing to the number of breasts on the human body" (73).

The addition of one or two extra appointments may not seem too onerous, and, indeed, for some it is a small price to pay for the opportunity to catch cancer early or to avoid risk-reducing surgeries; but as many of the women I interviewed explained, as the appointments pile up, the year becomes divided into smaller and smaller chunks of time—four-, three-, or even two-month intervals—when they feel somewhat normal. And, again, those four to seven appointments a year do not include follow-up scans and biopsies. But because no cancer-screening test is sensitive enough to catch every case of cancer and yet specific enough to avoid false positives, many BRCA+ women end up having some form of follow-up screening during their lifetimes. Hannah highlighted the toll that follow-up appointments can take: "It's so time consuming. It's like Monday you have a mammogram. They call you on Friday and they tell you they need more scans. Then you go back the next week for an MRI and then it's ultrasound but they can't do those on the same day. It has to be separate days and separate appointments. Each appointment takes three hours and by the time you're done, you can't work. You go home and sit on the couch and cry."

Here, again, we can see what a messy object we're dealing with. When enacted in the mode of screening, BRCA risk is dispersed over space and time, and the reason for this dispersal doesn't really have anything to do with risk per se. Rather, the dispersal has to do with *cancer*, with the practicalities of how and where cancer screening is performed. One episode of screening can mean multiple tests, over multiple days, weeks, or months, across multiple physical sites. And there is never just one episode. The need to screen for cancer never goes away but instead constantly recurs, creating a cycle that Stark described as "the yearly medical gauntlet" (105). To be sure, there are moments of intense relief within this cycle, and women who can get their results on-site the same day tend to feel that screening is more sustainable over the long term. But for other BRCA+ women, the routine of screening never really allows the threat of cancer to recede. Gessen wrote that it made her feel like a professional patient, like someone who would be considered ill until proven healthy and then, within just a month or two, would have to prove it all over again (74).

Reading the At-Risk Body: Breast MRI and the Problem
of False Positive Test Results

Proving one's health is not necessarily an easy task for a BRCA+ woman. It certainly wasn't for Gessen, whose first MRI found something suspicious and led to a breast biopsy. When the results of the biopsy came back negative, Gessen asked her doctor to stop treating her like a cancer patient since she did not, in fact, have cancer. Her doctor's response was to clarify that she had "no *detectable* cancer" (74; emphasis added). Such a response might seem cruel, like an unnecessary undermining of Gessen's confidence or a paranoid fear about a false negative in the face of pathological evidence to the contrary—and maybe it was. But I would argue that it is also a reflection of how cancer-screening practices enact or "do" the at-risk body. This is the claim that I made earlier, that when enacted in the mode of screening, the at-risk body is turned into a source of knowledge about cancer. Here I want to elaborate that claim and amend it slightly to say that within screening the at-risk body is turned into an *uncertain* or *equivocal* source of knowledge about cancer. That is, the at-risk body must be made readable so that physicians can know if its cells have produced a malignancy, but in this mode of enactment, the at-risk body is hard to read. Importantly, this is not to say that the at-risk body is inherently or naturally hard to read. Rather my point is just the opposite, namely that the practices that compose this mode of enactment make the body this way, and, as a result, the realities of risk and disease overlap.

That ovarian cancer–screening practices make the at-risk body hard to read is hardly debatable. Although there have been some recent developments in how CA-125 blood tests can be better used to detect ovarian cancer, the current medical consensus is that no form of screening effectively detects the disease at an early stage.[10] For this reason (as well as space constraints), I am going to focus my discussion here on breast cancer screening—on showing how even though it is an effective way of managing BRCA risk (or, rather, *because* it is an effective way of managing BRCA risk), it turns the at-risk body into an uncertain or equivocal source of knowledge about cancer. To do that, I'll briefly explain some of the history surrounding breast cancer screening for high-risk women, focusing specifically on the addition of breast MRI to the NCCN recommendations in 2009. I will then turn to the problem of false positive test results with breast MRI, arguing that they affect the actual reality of BRCA risk, not just a women's subjective perception of it. To support this argument I will turn to discourse from the FORCE message boards and other biosocial sources, but I will rely most heavily on clinical descriptions of the three main follow-up methods for false positive test results: short-interval screening, second-look ultrasound, and biopsy.

The idea that BRCA+ women can effectively manage breast cancer risk through screening is a relatively new one. When the BRCA mutations were discovered in the mid-1990s, clinicians could recommend two courses of action to BRCA+ women: risk-reducing bilateral mastectomy or an intensive surveillance regimen of monthly breast self-exams beginning at age eighteen, semiannual clinical breast exams beginning at age twenty-five, and annual mammograms beginning at age twenty-five (Lehman and Smith 1109). It soon became clear, though, that this regimen was inadequate, as mammography had only about 50 percent sensitivity in this population of high-risk women.[11] This low sensitivity rate meant false negatives or, in other words, missed cancers. Researchers attributed the low sensitivity of mammography in BRCA+ women in large part to the problem of breast density. Because women with BRCA mutations are more likely than women in the general population to develop breast cancer young, screening had to begin early, by age twenty-five according to the NCCN guidelines. But young women have denser breasts, meaning they have more of the fibroglandular tissue that images as white on a mammogram, potentially hiding malignant lesions, which also image as white. In addition, BRCA1-related cancers often appear benign in mammograms, showing up as "cellular and fleshy" masses with smooth, round margins rather than the more typical irregular or spiculated margins associated with malignancy (Dent and Warner 393). These problems of detection were confounded by the fact that breast cancers in young women (and especially in BRCA1 mutation carriers) tend to have shorter doubling times, which means they grow faster. Thus, when cancers were missed by mammogram and diagnosed later as interval cancers, they were more likely to be larger than 1 centimeter and to have already spread to lymph nodes (Raikhlin et al. 889).

Faced with the possibility that mammography was doing more harm than good in this high-risk population, researchers began looking for screening alternatives in the late 1990s and early 2000s. MRI was quickly identified as the most promising option, with numerous single and multisite trials demonstrating higher sensitivity than that of mammography or ultrasound. A 2009 review of ten such studies, for instance, found that the sensitivity rates of MRI ranged from 71 percent to 100 percent, which was considerably higher than the 13- to 59-percent range of mammography and the 13-to 65-percent range of ultrasound (Lehman 1110). In all of these studies, the higher sensitivity of MRI led to a cancer yield rate that almost doubled that of mammography screening alone (1110).

Researchers attributed these gains in sensitivity to several features of MRI, the main one being that the images it produces are not affected by breast density. In a mammogram, dense breast tissue appears white because it absorbs more ionizing radiation than fatty tissue. But MRIs don't rely on ionizing radiation to produce images. Rather, MRI images are based on how hydrogen atoms in the body realign themselves when radio waves are sent through a magnetic field that surrounds the patient. Depending on tissue type, the atoms emit different signals during the realignment process, allowing a computer to produce detailed, cross-sectional images of various tissue structures in the breast ("Breast Magnetic Resonance Imaging (MRI)"). In addition to how various structures look, however, MRI can also provide information about how they behave. It does this through the use of a contrast agent. After the MRI has produced an initial set of images, patients are injected with a contrast agent (usually gadolinium), and the rate at which different kinds of tissue absorb and release that agent is measured. This information, called the kinetic curve or contrast uptake and washout pattern, allows for further differentiation between benign and malignant lesions since the latter tend to absorb and release the contrast dye more quickly than the former (Dent and Warner 394). Specifically, there are three patterns of behavior a lesion (which can be a very small focus of enhancement, a mass, or a non-mass-like enhancement) might exhibit: (1) persistently enhancing; (2) plateau; and (3) washout. Persistently enhancing lesions show slow and gradual enhancement and are usually indicative of a benign condition. Those that show a plateau pattern enhance a great deal in the first couple of minutes but then slow down, indicating either a benign or malignant finding. The last of these curves, the washout curve, is the most indicative of malignancy, a fact that Dr. Barrett explained by saying that cancers are "hungry" but also "leaky" because they "have faulty cell membranes." In other words, "a cancer will take up contrast very rapidly, but then it leaks, so it goes down and washes out, and that's your classic type III malignant curve."

With the superiority of MRI as means of detecting breast cancer established, the American Cancer Society added the test to their screening guidelines for high-risk women in 2007, and the NCCN followed in 2009. The addition of breast MRI did not make screening a perfect way to manage BRCA-related breast cancer risk, but it did mean there was an "ethically justifiable" alternative to mastectomy, as along as the women who chose it could tolerate the small but not insignificant risk of a false negative (Dent and Warner 392, 399). But it wasn't just risk of false negatives that these high-risk women would have to tolerate. While breast MRI is the most sensitive breast cancer-screening test available, it is also the least specific, which means it identifies as suspicious more noncancerous lesions than mammography or ultrasound, resulting in a higher rate of false positives. Dr. Barrett described this problem of low specificity in terms of a "be careful what you wish for" scenario. With MRI, he explained, "you're very likely going to find something that you didn't know you were going to have to deal with, and then you've got to find a way to deal with it. I cringe when I see them coming, and I just hope that it's straightforward—[that] it's either obviously good or obviously bad, nothing in between." The frequency of "in between" MRI results, that is, those requiring callbacks for additional diagnostic testing, has been the subject of many studies. A 2006 *JAMA* study, for instance, found that the probability of additional testing after an initial or baseline MRI was 32 percent. That percentage dropped for subsequent MRIs but only to 20 percent (Plevritis et al. 2377). When the ACS published their updated screening guidelines for high-risk women in 2007, they noted that in all studies to date, MRI had significantly lower specificity rates than mammography, resulting in high call back rates for the test, with some community practices reporting callback rates as high as 50 percent (Saslow et al. 81–82). And more recently, a 2015 study of 650 high-risk women undergoing surveillance found that MRI led to more callbacks than mammography (119 and 13, respectively), as well as more breast biopsies (95 versus 19) (Raikhlin et al. 889).

Despite general dissatisfaction with breast MRI callback rates, these studies of test sensitivity and specificity often end on a hopeful note, as researchers look toward a future when false positive rates will be lower because of improved techniques and more experience on the part of radiologists. Until that time, though, they are willing to accept the lower specificity of MRI as a justifiable tradeoff for fewer false negatives (Saslow et al. 82). Based on the fact that more BRCA+ women choose screening than risk-reducing surgery, it would seem that they also think this tradeoff is justified—and why wouldn't they? False positives are not as bad as false negatives; they can't kill you or make you sick or require you to undergo chemotherapy for a cancer that could have been treated with surgery alone. False positives are, quite literally, a problem that BRCA+ women can live with. In some sense, though, that is precisely the point—BRCA+ women *live with* false positives, meaning that their effects can extend beyond individual instances and episodes of screening, producing in the women who have to deal with them (and in the clinicians who treat them) a sense that they have "busy breasts" or that despite getting the all clear, something malignant is "hiding" and will eventually cause problems.[12] Over the course of my research, I came to think of this predicament as an incredibly ironic one. MRI is supposed to give BRCA+ women more assurance that they don't have cancer—that a negative result is truly a negative result. But going through the experience of a false positive, as so many BRCA+ women do, can undermine this assurance, making it easy to think that something malignant is actually there, and the imaging just hasn't found it yet.

This point is borne out in the FORCE message boards, particularly in threads where women share troublesome test results in order to get advice and solace from those who have had similar experiences.[13] While the details of such posts differ, they tend to exhibit a common pattern, beginning with the initial report of a suspicious finding, moving next to the ordeal of follow-up, and then ending with news of a benign (or sometimes indeterminate) result. Insofar as no one wants malignant results, news of a benign or indeterminate result always brings relief. But over time—whether it's the time between tests in one false positive scare or the time between separate false positives—the meaning of a benign result can change, indicating not that one has no cancer but rather, as

Gessen's doctor put it, one has no *detectable* cancer. Take, for example, the experience described in "Trying not to freak out," a FORCE message board thread started by a BRCA1+ woman who was concerned about the results of her regular screening MRI. A letter from her doctor's office indicated that she needed "further evaluation." Fearful and frustrated by the lack of information, she posted on the message board in order to get support from women who had been through similar ordeals. After others chimed in with their experiences, the original poster wrote back to report that a call to her doctor's office revealed that they wanted to do an MRI-guided biopsy on a "a small area that looks suspicious, which did not show up last year." After the biopsy, she posted to say that they "could not find the area that lit up on the MRI last time," and so she was told "it's a good sign that it disappeared" and to return in six months for follow-up. After others again chimed in with similar stories, she ended the thread with a final post about the cumulative effect of screening. "I'm starting to lose count of the number of mammograms, ultrasounds, MRIs, and biopsies I've had. [...] It's more than ten, and yet they haven't found anything that's clearly a problem yet; just a lot of areas to watch. Sigh."

It's important to point out that when it comes to this problem of false positives and the way they can turn the breast into a set of "areas to watch," researchers have done more than just hope for a better future. Since the early 2000s, when MRI was identified as a necessary supplement to mammography, dozens of studies have been conducted in order to understand the effects of false positives on women at high risk of breast cancer. What counts as an "effect" in such studies, though, is limited to a woman's subjective perception of her cancer risk, which is almost always understood in contrast to her real or "objective" cancer risk. For instance, a fifty-year-old woman with a BRCA2 mutation has about a 37 percent chance of developing breast cancer (Bougie and Weberpals 2), but the concern in these studies is that false positives could cause her to overestimate that risk by repeatedly reminding her of her high-risk status, thus enhancing her cancer worry.[14] To be sure, this concern is well founded, and I think it's important to pay attention to the reasons why many women, not just BRCA+ women, overestimate their breast cancer risk.[15] But by identifying reality with "objective" cancer risk (that is, a lifetime risk assessment) and paying attention to false positives only insofar as they affect its counterpart—subjective risk perception—such studies leave little room for considering how false positives themselves are a way of producing reality. Yes, BRCA+ women react emotionally to the tests that tell them they might have cancer, and comments like those above from the FORCE message boards can tell us something about those reactions, but they can also tell us something about BRCA risk, about what it *is* when enacted by cancer-screening practices and about how those practices put the at-risk body in question, making it an uncertain or equivocal source of knowledge about cancer and thus allowing risk and disease to overlap.

To some degree, that idea that cancer-screening practices put the at-risk body in question is self-evident. Any cancer-screening finding, whether it ends up benign or malignant, has the potential to undermine what we know about our bodies and our health, at least for a period of time. *Something is there, but is it actually cancer?* The problem with MRI-detected findings is that answering this question can be an arduous process, one that some BRCA+ women have described in terms of the ups and downs of a roller coaster.[16] As is the case with mammography and ultrasound, MRI-detected findings are assigned a score of 0 to 6 according to the Breast Imaging, Reporting, and Data System (BI-RADS), which is a standardized lexicon and scoring scale that was developed by the American College of Radiology in the 1990s.[17] With the exception of a 6, which is assigned to biopsy-proven malignancies, these scores do not indicate if a finding is cancer. Rather, BI-RADs scores for breast MRI are interpretations of information (morphology and kinetics) that radiologists use to sort findings into categories and to indicate what should happen next. In other words, BI-RADS scores determine *how*—through what method—the "Is it actually cancer?" question will be answered. But each of these three methods can, itself, be a source of ambiguity even as it is deployed as a means of eliminating ambiguity. Below I describe these three methods—short-interval follow-up, second-look screening, and breast biopsy—in order to show how, through a number of practical, logistical, and technological limitations, they can enact the at-risk body as an uncertain or equivocal source of knowledge about cancer. Although I have tried to make these descriptions detailed, I have not been able to make them comprehensive, which is to say they do not include every possible scenario that might arise because of a breast MRI finding. Yet even still, I think it's easy to see why Dr. Barrett would say that he "cringes" when he sees a breast MRI coming his way and, relatedly, why BRCA+ women would compare the experience of high-risk breast cancer screening to being on a roller coaster.

A Roller Coaster of Follow-Ups

Of the seven BI-RADS designations a radiologist can assign to an MRI finding, three require follow-up because of concern about malignancy: BI-RADS 3, 4, and 5. Of those three designations, BI-RADS 3 indicates the lowest level of concern—that the lesion is "probably benign" and that the follow-up (that is, the means of answering the "Is it actually cancer?" question) should be short-interval screening, usually another MRI six months later. In order for a radiologist to categorize a finding as BI-RADS 3 and make this recommendation, he or she must believe it has no more than a 2 percent chance of being malignant. So, when the BI-RADS descriptor for this category says "probably benign," that is what it means: findings placed in this category should very rarely lead to a cancer diagnosis. In fact, according to the American College of Radiology BI-RADS Atlas, a criterion for recommending short-interval follow-up is that the radiologist does not expect the findings to change over the six-month period. Short-interval follow-up, then, is a way to establish lesion stability before recommending a return to routine screening. Contrary to how it might sound, though, this is not a particularly quick way of answering the "Is it really cancer?" question. Establishing lesion stability is a two- or three-year process that begins with the follow-up MRI six months after the initial BI-RADS 3 score. If the lesion is stable at this scan, then another BI-RADS 3 score is given, along with a recommendation for another six-month follow-up MRI. Then, at this one-year mark, if there is no change, the lesion again receives a BI-RADS 3 score but this time with a recommendation for one-year follow-up. At this point—two years from the initial finding—the radiologist can downgrade the score to a BI-RADS 2 (which indicates a benign finding) or continue for one more year at a BI-RADS 3 (Morris et al. 140).

Despite how long it can take, the obvious advantage to this "wait and see" approach is that it provides patients with a less invasive, less painful, and less expensive alternative to immediate biopsy. Relatively speaking, then, short-interval follow-up is perceived to be a low-stakes way of answering the "Is it really cancer?" question. Because of this perception, though, and because there are no specific criteria for determining what counts as a BI-RADS 3 on MRI (Lourenco et al. 1037; Leung, "Utility of Second-Look Ultrasound" 272), short-interval follow-up is also an overused intervention (Eby et al. 865), with some studies showing that as many as one in three women undergoing breast MRI will be called back for subsequent imaging (Eby et al., "Probably Benign" 310). In this sense, the BI-RADS 3 designation can act as a "holding tank" for question-able lesions, especially when radiologists have little experience or when there are no previous MRIs for comparison (Rylands-Monk 13; Eby et al. 866; Morris et al. 138; Liberman et al. 378). On the one hand, we might argue (and some researchers have) that this overuse of BI-RADS 3 is not a problem because the cancer yield rate is consistently very low, which means that in addition to being a less invasive, less painful, and less expensive alternative to biopsy, short-interval follow-up is a "safe alternative to biopsy" (Eby et al. 865). On the other hand, though, if we are interested in understanding how screening practices make the at-risk body hard to read, then we might argue that this overuse is a problem *precisely because* of the low cancer yield rate. That might seem like a strange way to put it, and I certainly don't mean to suggest that this situation would some-how be better if more MRI-detected BI-RADS 3 lesions turned out to be malignant. That the great majority of these lesions are eventually determined to be stable and therefore benign is obviously a good thing. But determining a lesion as benign does not make it go away. The lesion is there now: screening has identified it, put it on the map, so to speak, and made it part of the breast, made it, as Dr. Barrett put it, something that must be dealt with, even if that just means waiting six months to see if it changes. Lizzy Stark recounted her reac-tion to this situation in *Pandora's DNA*, explaining that as she read the BI-RADS 3 result on her mammogram report, she thought to herself "Probably benign. Probably. The thing in my breast was probably benign. Chances were really good that it was nothing. But probably benign isn't the same as benign. So, they did find something. Something that was probably nothing, but still something. There was something in my breast" (180).

When radiologists are not comfortable watching something that is probably benign but feel that immediate biopsy is not warranted, they can try to answer the "Is it actually cancer?" question with targeted or "second-look" screening, which is almost always done by ultrasound. Ultrasound is the preferred method for targeted screening because it is relatively easy to perform, does not require an IV for administering a contrast agent, is well tolerated by patients, and does not expose them to radiation, as mammography does (Hollowell et al. 1282). Yet despite these advantages, the usefulness of targeted ultrasound after MRI is a debated topic in the world of breast imaging. The ACR BI-RADS Atlas notes that there are no established guidelines for who should have ultrasound after MRI (Morris et al. 141), and multiple studies have demonstrated that its use varies widely among radiologists (Hollowell et al. 1279; Leung, "Utility of

Second-Look Ultrasound" 261). Probably the most straightforward use of targeted ultrasound after MRI is in the case of a BI-RADS 0 score, which indicates that the exam was inconclusive and additional imaging is needed before the radiologist can make any recommendations (Morris et al. 137). Targeted ultrasound can also provide additional diagnostic information in the case of BI-RADS 3 scores, although this is a less "thoroughly established use" of the technology (Leung, "Second-Look Ultrasound" S87). The idea here is that a second look with ultrasound can allow the radiologist to either confirm the "probably benign" nature of the lesion or revise the score down to a 2 (which means it is confirmed benign and routine screening is recommended) or up to a 4 (which means it is suspicious for malignancy and biopsy is recommended), thereby obviating the need to wait six months for follow-up.

What makes this use (or any use, really) of targeted ultrasound after MRI questionable is the problem of correlation or, in other words, the problem of confirming that the ultrasound-detected lesion is the same as the MRI-detected lesion. Ultrasound and MRI produce images in very different ways, the former through sound waves with patients in the supine, oblique, or lateral decubitus positions and the latter through magnetic resonance imaging with patients in the prone position (Leung, "Utility of Second-Look Ultrasound" 261). Translating information about lesion size and location from one modality to the other, then, is difficult, requiring radiologists to establish correlation according to other features, namely lesion shape and "concordance in probability of malignancy," which means that if one image looks suspicious for cancer and the other doesn't, then the radiologist needs to assume there is no correlation (262). In only about half of the targeted ultrasounds performed, though, will correlation even be a possibility. Numerous studies have demonstrated that the chance of an MRI-detected lesion showing up on ultrasound is around 50 percent, and that those lesions that do show up are more likely to be large, to be identified on MRI as a mass or focus (as opposed to a non-mass-like enhancement), and to be malignant (Leung, "Utility of Second-Look Ultrasound" 266–69; Dall 1123). What's interesting (or troubling, rather) about this last feature is that while malignant lesions do show up better on ultrasound than benign lesions, they often show up *as* benign lesions, that is, as "nonspecific and subtle—without malignant characteristics" (Abe et al. 375). Hence the concern over using targeted ultrasound in BI-RADS 3 cases: the possibility that something malignant could be downgraded to 2 or watched for six months.

Difficulties with lesion correlation also come into play with the third and final means of answering the "Is it actually cancer?" question—biopsy. Breast biopsy is the management recommendation when the radiologist believes there is more than a 2 percent chance that a finding is malignant. If the chance of malignancy is assessed to be somewhere between 3 percent and 95 percent, then the finding is categorized as BI-RADS 4, "suspicious for malignancy." If the chance of malignancy is assessed to be greater than 95 percent, then the finding is categorized as BI-RADS 5, "highly suggestive of malignancy." As these percentages indicate, the threshold for performing biopsy on an MRI finding is low; all that's required is for the radiologist to determine that the lesion has a 3 percent or greater chance of being malignant. Once that determination has been made, he or she can proceed either with a needle biopsy, which means making a small incision in the breast and removing tissue samples through a hollow, sometimes vacuum-assisted needle, or with a surgical biopsy, which means removing either the entire lesion or part of it though open surgical procedure.

Because they are less invasive, less costly, and allow for better treatment planning in the case of a cancer diagnosis, needle biopsies are performed more often than open surgical biopsies; thus my discussion here will focus on that method. However, elements of that discussion (namely those that deal with the issue of correlation) apply to surgical biopsies as well, since most biopsies of MRI-detected lesions, whether surgical or needle, are by necessity image-guided biopsies.[18] The great advantage of MRI is that it can detect lesions long before they are palpable. But if a lesion cannot be felt, it must be located through some kind of radiologic imaging before it can be biopsied. Any facility that performs breast MRI should have the ability to do MRI-guided biopsies, but that procedure is not typically a radiologist's first choice. As I will explain in more detail below, MRI-guided biopsies are difficult to perform and resource intensive, requiring considerable time and technical expertise. In most cases, then, a radiologist will perform a targeted ultrasound, hoping that if the lesion shows up, an ultrasound-guided biopsy can be performed. The features that make ultrasound-guided biopsy preferable to MRI-guided biopsy are, for the most part, the same ones that make ultrasound the preferred means of "second-look" screening: it's relatively easy to perform, it's better tolerated by patients, and it doesn't require an IV for contrast agent or expose them to radiation (Leung, "Utility of Second-Look Ultrasound" 260; Mahoney and Newell 17).

In addition, though, ultrasound-guided biopsy allows for real-time visualiza-tion of the lesion, meaning that after the target spot has been identified and a biopsy needle is inserted, the radiologist can use ultrasound to confirm that the needle is the right location and watch its path as it is "fired into the lesion" in order to retrieve tissue samples (Mahoney and Newell 19).

As noted earlier, though, about 50 percent of the time the lesion is not going to show up on ultrasound. And while having a lesion show up (even if it looks benign) can be confirmation of the need to biopsy, the converse is not true: lack of ultrasound finding does not diminish the need to biopsy a BI-RADS 4 or 5 lesion. Rather, it means that the biopsy will need to be MRI-guided rather than ultrasound guided (Leung, "Utility of Second-Look Ultrasound" 269; Chopier et al. 214; Hollowell et al. 1283). The difficulty of MRI-guided biopsy stems, in part, from the fact that most MRI machines are still closed, which means that in order for the radiologist to see the lesion, the patients must be *inside* the machine. But in order for the radiologist to biopsy the lesion, the patient must be *outside* the machine. Thus, in MRI-guided breast biopsy, there is no real-time viewing and sampling of the lesion (Chopier et al. 216). Rather, these steps must happen separately. In brief (and truly, this is only a summary of the process), this is done by first positioning the patient's breast between two compression plates, one of which is a grid that maps the breast and guides needle placement at the time of biopsy. Once an IV is in place for administering the contrast agent, the patient is shuttled in and out of the MRI machine for imaging three or four times, as the area of concern is identified on the MRI and mapped to a location in the breast. Then, once the patient is outside of the machine, that location is marked by inserting a device called an "obturator" into the breast. That mark is then checked by imaging, and the patient is shuttled out again and the biopsy is performed. Finally, a titanium clip is inserted into the biopsy cavity and that location is once again checked on MRI—all while the patient is lying prone, as still as possible, on the imaging table (Mahoney and Newell 20–21). In facilities where MRI-guided biopsies are done frequently, this process might take about an hour. But in facilities like Dr. Barrett's, where they have the equip-ment and capacity for MRI-guided biopsies but don't perform many, the process is "very laborious and cumbersome." "Without the proper experience and with-out an experienced technologist who is really good at it, to streamline it, it could take two or three hours." And in the end "you may not even be that convinced you got representative tissue."

This concern over getting "representative tissue" is, of course, a concern over correlation, but in this case, it's not correlation between imaging modalities, for example, ultrasound and MRI. Instead it's correlation between the first MRI images that prompted the biopsy and the subsequent images produced at the time of biopsy in order to relocate the suspicious area. Correlating breast images produced at different times by any one screening modality could be difficult for a number of reasons, such as hormone-related breast changes, differences in patient positioning, and differences in imaging technique and/or technician. But the task is particularly challenging with MRI because images are produced by the uptake of the contrast agent, and the rate of that uptake can easily be affected by the compression plates used to hold the breast in place and guide the needle (which are not needed during a regular screening MRI). If the compression plates are too tight, then "vascularization" within the lesion will be reduced, resulting in less uptake and a different image (Chopier et al. 216). If the compression plates are not tight enough, then the breast can move, and, again, the image will be different. Yet even if the plates don't interfere, correlation can remain difficult because what is, in part, used to identify the lesion—the uptake of the contrast agent—is not constant over time but rather drops off after injection, making the image transitory (217, 222). Unlike ultrasound-guided biopsy, then, there's no way for the radiologist to confirm in real-time if he or she has sampled the right tissue. That confirmation can only come later, when the pathologist analyzes the sample and determines if there is a match between its histological features and the MRI images (218). If there is a match—either suspicious images with malignant histology or probably benign images with benign histology—then presumably the "Is it actually cancer?" question has been answered. In the latter case, though, the patient will most likely have a follow-up MRI six months later to establish lesion stability (220). In cases where there is no match between imaging and histology, then maybe the "Is it actually cancer?" question has been answered, and maybe it hasn't. If the imaging says probably benign, but the histology says malignant, then the assumption is that the patient has cancer, but the pathology will need to be confirmed and the images reviewed to determine what suspicious features, if any, were missed. If the images say suspicious but the histology says benign, then, in some cases, the patient might not have cancer but rather a benign lesion that mimics cancer, for example, a granular cell tumor, sclerosing adenosis, or fat necrosis. In other cases, though, when no specific benign condition is identified (and in some cases, even when it is), the radiologist will have to consider the possibility that the area of concern was not properly targeted and sampled and that, therefore, another biopsy, possibly a surgical biopsy, is needed (221).

This problem of correlation in MRI-guided biopsy looms large in the world of high-risk breast cancer screening, and it's easy to see why. If a radiologist samples the wrong tissue in an MRI-guided biopsy, and the pathologist incorrectly determines that the suspect lesion is benign, then it could be six months to a year before that lesion is seen again, and that's if the patient follows the recommended screening regimen. In the case of a fast-growing breast cancer (for instance, the kind of triple negative breast cancer associated with BRCA1 mutations), six months can mean the difference between curable and incurable disease. It is not an overstatement, then, to say that nothing less than life itself is at stake in the possibility of a false negative. What I have tried to show here, though, is that there is also something at stake in the possibility of a false positive and, further, that this something cannot be understood only or even primarily in terms of a woman's subjective perception of her risk, which stands in contrast to her real, "objective" risk. False positives themselves are a way of producing reality. The combined high sensitivity and low specificity of breast MRI means that it will "find everything," as women on the FORCE message boards often put it, and "finding everything" is a way of populating the breast, of mapping its interior and putting the at-risk body in question as an uncertain or equivocal source of knowledge about cancer. This uncertainty would not be so significant if there were easier, more reliable ways to answer the "Is it actually cancer?" question. But often answering that question is a process, one that is not governed by strict or clear guidelines and one where each option a radiologist might choose as a means of follow-up brings with it as much potential for enhancing uncertainty as it does for diminishing it.

Living Under the Sword of Damocles

Given this potential for uncertainty, is it any wonder that a BRCA+ woman might say that her breasts are "busy," that she feels something is "hiding" in them, or—worse—that she is "living under the sword of Damocles," as though getting breast cancer is "more of a when than an if." These last two comments were made by Nancy, the fifty-six-year-old technical writer whose awkward experience with an oncologist I recounted earlier in this chapter. Nancy's reference to Damocles' sword echoes many similarly deterministic comments made within the biosocial communities surrounding BRCA risk. In blogs, op-eds, and memoirs, BRCA+ women often say they feel like their risk is a "ticking time bomb" or that they're playing "Russian roulette." Using the rhetorical methodology deployed by scholars like Happe, Crabb and LeCouteur, and Dubriwny, we might argue that such language is evidence of the type of overlap between risk and disease that results from (and propagates) ideologies of genetic determinism. We might further argue that it indexes the failure of BRCA+ women to understand—and thus of the medical establishment to explain—the fact that BRCA mutations do not carry 100 percent penetrance. No woman with a BRCA mutation is destined to get breast or ovarian cancer. There are no metaphorical swords hanging over their heads, no time bombs in their chests, no loaded guns pointed at their heads. But there are hands that palpate the lumps and thickenings of their breasts, machines that identify "areas of concern" and produce images of them, grids that map breasts, compression plates that hold them in place, and needles that vacuum tissue samples out of them. Can we try to understand this deterministic language in relation to the physicalities of practices like these and the realities they produce, acknowledging, as Condit did in 1999, that to do so is not to deny the creativity of language by reducing it to physical matter but rather to appreciate more fully how meaning arises materially through the interaction of language with a "social-material universe that resists our rearrangement of it" ("The Materiality of Coding" 333, 335)? If not, then I worry that we risk making the same troubling move that studies of the effects of false positives have made—that of prioritizing "subjective" perception of cancer risk in such a way and to such a degree that all we count as "objective" reality are the supposedly "mute facts" of science. Only in our case, those "mute facts" would then become the fodder of critique, and "subjective" wouldn't refer to the kind of psychologized notion of selfhood implied in those false positive studies but rather to the discourses that make up the subject, constituting her as a patient without symptoms, a responsible citizen, a self-sacrificing mother, or any number of other subject positions that cause her to overestimate her cancer risk. To be sure, these two versions of "subjective" are very different, and they obviously lead to different kinds of analysis. But for all of their differences, they are, as Andreas Reckwitz has put it, "secret allies" when it comes to the status of the material world, a world that they both leave untouched insofar as the objects populating it exist only in terms of how a subject knows them (202).

BRCA risk, though, is not just something that BRCA+ women know. As I hope that I have begun to demonstrate here, it is also something that they *do*, and through this doing it comes to have a reality in their lives. In the case of high-risk breast cancer–screening practices, that reality overlaps with the reality of disease, as breasts are repeatedly palpated, scanned, imaged, compressed, and sampled. For Hannah, this regimen had such a negative effect on her quality of life that she eventually decided to have risk-reducing bilateral mastectomy. People who questioned her decision correctly pointed out that there was a decent chance she would have never been diagnosed with breast cancer. Her simple response—"But my life will still be ruined by it"—trenchantly captures my point here. Screening enacts BRCA risk through an ensemble of practices, instruments, techniques, and technologies designed to detect *cancer*. Thus, the at-risk body is turned into a source of knowledge about *cancer*. This is a real overlap between risk and disease, one that we can explain but not one that we can explain away. It is, as Mol would say, a tension in medicine ("Proving or Improving" 411). BRCA+ women and their physicians want fewer false negatives, but outside of risk-reducing surgery, this means dealing with more false positives, and, as I have tried to show here, this tradeoff has serious consequences, not the least of which is the uncertainty and ambiguity that comes with trying to make the at-risk body readable. But—and this caveat is essential—*it is an entirely reasonable and justifiable tradeoff*. It makes sense. In fact, it makes so much sense that we might say that women who don't want to have risk-reducing surgery, don't have a lot of choice here. They feel intense pressure to choose MRI, despite the problems it creates. This is a real constraint, one that impinges greatly on the freedom of BRCA+ women. But this lack of freedom does not call for emancipation. It does not call, in other words, for another rhetoric of choice. The lack of freedom that BRCA+ women experience, no matter what health-care practices (if any) they participate in, calls for a rhetoric of care, and so it is to that subject, care, and how we might foster a rhetoric of it, that I now turn.

4

Toward a Rhetoric of Care for the At Risk

As I noted in the introduction to this book, I do not believe that I (or anyone else) can just create a rhetoric of care for the at risk. A real rhetoric of care can emerge only over time, just as rhetorics of choice have done over decades of debates within and about genetic medicine. But that doesn't mean there's nothing we can do to hasten its emergence. Our thinking about genetic risk is so saturated by choice that even to talk about care in this context would count as a step in the right direction. However, what I aim to offer here is somewhat more specific than the suggestion that we need to talk about care. Taking a page from Richard McKeon's book, my goal here is to use rhetoric architectonically, offering "discoveries" that I have made through my engagements with BRCA-related discourses as "places by which to perceive creatively what might otherwise not be experienced in the existent world we constitute" (14–15). I am well aware that for a project that takes its inspiration from the ontological turn, the idea of using rhetoric architectonically might come across as a contradictory move. I will address this issue later, but for now the more important (but related) point I want to highlight is that this task, to "perceive creatively," is somewhat different from the purpose that rhetorical commonplaces usually serve within RSTM scholarship, where a set of topoi often acts as an interpretive device or what Prelli refers to as "a fertile vantage point from which to understand the rhetoric that goes on in any substantive field" (73). The topics I offer here fit this bill somewhat, but their primary purpose is different than the one described by Prelli. With them, I don't aim to explain what is happening in this "substantive field" as much as I aim to change it.[1] To be sure, this is a tricky distinction, and there are times when I fail to maintain it, but nevertheless, I believe that it makes sense to identify my mode of engagement here with invention rather than interpretation. Rhetorics of choice are pervasive in the biosocial discourses of BRCA+ women. In those discourses, we hear a constant refrain about the necessity of personal choice and the gift of empowerment through knowledge.

But rather than interpreting what we know is already there (and showing why so much of it is an illusion), we need to invent something new, to offer the participants an arena in which to gather. While I don't claim that the four topics I present in this chapter are any kind of panacea for the problems created by an overreliance on choice in discourses surrounding BRCA risk, I do think they can help build these arenas. After all, what are topics if not rhetorical arenas in which to gather?

Orientations

Before I get to those topics, however, I want to examine this relationship between interpretation and invention and, through that examination, to articulate a theoretical framework for what I am trying to do here. Earlier in the book I acknowledged that my goal of extending Mol's work into the domain of genetic risk could be seen as an ethically fraught task because of its potential to further muddy the line between health and illness that has troubled genetic medicine for decades. But it could also be seen as a theoretically fraught task insofar as it is based on a specious opposition between invention and interpretation, that is, between rhetoric's heuristic capacities and its hermeneutic capacities. On the one hand, this opposition is specious because the practices of inventing and interpreting are not easy to distinguish from each other. The simplest explanation of this practical inseparability comes from Schleiermacher, who argued that "every act of understanding is the reverse side of an act of speaking," thus providing us with the "two sides of the same coin" metaphor (quoted in Pullman 156). Rhetoric, on one side, creates meaning, and hermeneutics, on the other, extracts it. The two practices cannot be separated because the latter depends on the former. More recently, rhetorical hermeneutics (or hermeneutical rhetoric[2]) has provided us with a more complex explanation of this practical inseparability by showing how these practices mutually define each other. Rhetoric and hermeneutics cannot be separated in practice because, as Steven Mailloux put it, they are "practical forms of the same extended human activity." In order to produce rhetoric, we must interpret a situation, and to communicate an interpretation, we must produce rhetoric. Thus, for Mailloux, "hermeneutics is the rhetoric of establishing meaning and rhetoric is the hermeneutics of problematic linguistic situations (379).[3]

This practical inseparability is important to acknowledge, but it doesn't pose any real problem here. My own act of rhetorical invention certainly depends on my reading of a "problematic linguistic situation," but that doesn't mean that the product of that reading must then be used primarily as a way to interpret meaning. There is, however, another kind of inseparability at work, one that is more historical and philosophical in nature, and that does pose a problem. Simply put, this problem is that within rhetoric studies invention has provided the theoretical justification for precisely the kind of purification that I am trying to move away from. Here, I am referring to the eventual alignment of rhetoric—via the movement from a managerial to an epistemic view of invention—with antifoundationalism and social constructivism and the kind of rhetorical analysis that alignment led to. If rhetoric didn't just dress arguments but also invented them, the reasoning went, then arguments in any field (even science) could be understood in rhetorical terms.[4] Herbert Simons described this development in his introduction to *The Rhetorical Turn*, identifying the social constructivist view as one in which "[p]eople and places, problems and causes are all in effect 'created' by language" and arguing that according to this view, the job of the rhetorical analyst is, in part, "to determine how constructions of the 'real' are made persuasive" (11). Simons expressed some concern about this kind of rhetorical analysis by pointing out (following Woolgar and Pawluch) that it requires a good deal of "ontological gerrymandering," (11) but it was Dilip Gaonkar's critique seven years later in *Rhetorical Hermeneutics* that raised serious questions about rhetoric's ability to function as an interpretive tool, creating what Gross described as a "reflective moment in which to meditate on the methodological limitations of first generation rhetoric of science" (*Starring the Text* 14). In brief, Gaonkar's argument was that rhetoric's interpretive capacities were limited for three reasons: one, it was a primarily productive enterprise; two, it was agent centered; and three, it was thin, meaning it lacked the hermeneutic constraints necessary for fruitful interpretations. But also at issue for Gaonkar—and more relevant to the problems with purification that I've identified in this book—was the ubiquity of rhetoric and the sense that anything could be reduced to its function. Gaonkar believed that rhetoricians had been "seduced" by the "dream of interpretation," that is, the idea that as a kind of "hermeneutic metadiscourse" rhetoric could produce a "perfect interpretation" in which the objects under investigation lost all of their "recalcitrance" and became "transparent" (25). Having "entered the orbit of general hermeneutics," rhetoric was, according to this dream, a "way of reading the endless discursive debris that surrounded us" (25). "It is a habit of our time," Gaonkar argued disapprovingly, "to invoke rhetoric, time and again, to make sense of a wide variety of discursive practices that beset and perplex us, and of discursive artifacts that annoy and entertain us, and of discursive formations that inscribe and subjugate us" (25).

To return to the problem posed by this second kind of inseparability, then, we might say that if rhetoric did enter "the orbit of general hermeneutics" during this time, then it was invention that propelled it there. What began in the 1960s as an effort to expand the epistemic function of invention had helped produce, by the 1990s, a style of rhetorical analysis that saw science as rhetoric "without remainder," as Alan Gross so famously put it ("Origin of the Species" 107). And even though second and third generation rhetoric of science scholarship tended to back off such sweeping epistemological claims, we can still see the legacy of that expansion of invention in the work of rhetoricians like Happe and Dubriwny, where the object under investigation, BRCA risk, cannot help but lose its recalcitrance as it becomes part of the much larger operation of various cultural narratives and ideologies. If this is the case, then how can I claim invention as the way forward? That is, how can I offer invention as an alternative to precisely the kind of critique that it helped to foster? The short answer to this question is that I need a different version of invention, one that does not carry with it the epistemological implications that lead to constructivist critique. In some sense, this is a tricky request since historically speaking we have needed to understand invention as epistemic so that it wouldn't be understood as managerial. Within this binary, which has loomed very large in the history of rhetoric, a less epistemic version of invention has typically meant a less powerful version. As Janet Atwill has noted, though, binaries have never served invention very well. She made this point in reference to the oppositions between theory and practice, subjectivism and empiricism, and aestheticism and utilitarianism that have made it hard for this canon to find a home in American institutions of higher learning ("Finding a Home or Making a path" xi–xii). I would argue that it applies just as well to the opposition between managerial and epistemic views of invention. No matter where we place invention in relation to these two points, the question we are concerned with is a question about knowledge: *To what degree does rhetoric create knowledge?* We are well aware of the problems that accompany a conservative response to this question, one that places invention at the managerial end of the spectrum. But as so many in rhetoric and communication studies begin to organize their work around new materialist and ontological theories of rhetoric, it is becoming clear that we can't count on the opposite response, one that locates invention at the epistemic end of the spectrum, to continue providing this important concept with a sound or convincing theoretical justification. Without moving back into a managerial position, we need a version of invention that is nonepistemological in orientation, one that even if it's not built from new materialist and ontological theories of rhetoric, can at least accommodate them. In what follows, then, I try to indicate what such a non-epistemological orientation to invention might look like, focusing specifically on Richard McKeon's concept of an architectonic productive art, Atwill's interpretation of the ancient Greek concept of *logon techne*, and John Muckelbauer's related notions of affirmative repetition and productive reading. While these concepts are far from synonymous (and, in fact, are at odds with each other in some ways), I believe they can help provide the kind of theoretical framework that I need for fostering a rhetoric of care for the at risk.

Invention Outside Epistemology

If the aim here is to move away from a version of invention that focuses on questions of epistemology, then it is more than a little ironic that the first source I am going to turn to is Richard McKeon's 1971 "The Uses of Rhetoric in a Technological Age," a locus classicus for those who have wanted to explain and expand rhetoric's epistemic powers.[5] The essay was first published in *The Prospect of Rhetoric*, a book that helped considerably to spur the shift from a managerial to an epistemic view of invention. McKeon's contribution to this effort was to call for rhetoric to become, as it had been in the Roman Empire and the Renaissance, an architectonic productive art, meaning that its creative purview would not be limited to the content of verbal arguments but rather would extend to the production of schemata or devices that could guide the use of other arts (2, 12). For him, rhetoric was not about passively receiving the "data of existence" but instead about actively and creatively modifying that data in order to open up new avenues for action and to solve complex twentieth-century problems that were not distributed precisely in disciplines (17–18). Rhetoric was uniquely suited to these tasks, he believed, because its fields and methods transcended individual subject matters. McKeon focused on one of rhetoric's methods—the commonplaces—in particular, arguing that they should be used as "a means by which to light up modes and meanings of works of art and natural occurrences and to open up aspects and connections in existence and possibility" (14–15). In McKeon's view, commonplaces functioned more as a way of giving something presence (in Perelman and Olbrect-Tyteca's sense of that term) than as a way of generating content for an argument. As Hauser and Cushman put it, McKeon's view of the commonplaces transformed the aim of rhetoric from that of adherence or understanding to that of "making *selections* [. . .]. Rhetoric literally is the art of selecting conceptual starting-'places' or analytic categories which may be used efficaciously in thought/address that creates what are relevant matters and recognized facts" (220).

We usually think of rhetoric as the art of *using* conceptual starting places or analytic categories in order to engage in argument and produce knowledge. But here Hauser and Cushman have argued that for McKeon, rhetoric is the art of *selecting* conceptual starting places. Whether we deem the commonplaces epistemic or not, the use of them isn't what rhetoric—in McKeon's understanding—aims to do. Of course this distinction doesn't do much to counter the epistemological implications that have played out for decades in constructivist critique. Rhetoric might not be the use of conceptual starting places to create knowledge via argument, but by selecting or creating those conceptual starting places used by other arts in the creation of knowledge, it certainly retains a strong epistemic function. We can see this in the second part of the Hauser and Cushman quotation—"which may be used efficaciously in thought/address that creates what are relevant matters and recognized facts" (220). There is no way, then, to say that McKeon's work doesn't provide the justification for understanding rhetoric as a global hermeneutic. If rhetoric selects or creates the tool that is used elsewhere in the creation of knowledge, then that knowledge can be understood in rhetorical terms. We get the sense that by placings rhetoric in the superordinate position above all other arts as the dominant means of discovery, this is what McKeon intended, that rhetoric, not metaphysics, would be regarded as first philosophy (McKeon 18; Depew 37).

As justified as such a reading is, though, I believe it misses something about the nature of technics, namely that it is a kind of making or bringing forth whose products are meant to help their users *do* something rather than *know* something. Aristotle made this distinction in *Nicomachean Ethics*, in which he explained the three components of his tripartite theory of knowledge: *episteme* (theoretical knowledge), *techne* (productive knowledge), and *praxis* (practical knowledge). Both *techne* and *praxis* are concerned with the variable, that is, with those things not governed by nature or necessity, but whereas the end of *praxis*—*eudaimonia* or "the good life"—is inherently valuable, the end of *techne* is instrumentally valuable, abiding solely in the use of its product by a user. This instrumentality also distinguishes *techne* from *episteme*, which is an unchanging knowledge of first principles that cannot be applied in order to accomplish or produce anything (1140b31). Atwill further elaborated these distinctions in her 1998 *Rhetoric Reclaimed: Aristotle and the Liberal Arts Tradition*, a book that traces the forgotten features of *techne* through pre-Aristotelian texts in order to highlight its incompatibility with the "normalizing tendencies of the Western tradition of humanism" (7). Both *techne* and *episteme* operate according to various *logoi*, or reasoned accounts, she argued, but those of *techne*, unlike those of *episteme*, are "provisional explanations" designed to enable some kind of intervention in a particular place and at a particular time, not to provide users with any kind of lasting knowledge about the objects or practices with which they deal (98). In other words, we might say that the reasoned accounts of *techne* are like tools insofar as they do not represent or explain the problems they are meant to intervene into. Atwill turned to the *technai* of rhetoric and medicine in order to illustrate this point, arguing that neither the rhetorician nor the physician aimed to construct an account that simply "explained" a phenomenon in either discourse or healing. Rather, for them, the accounts of *techne* were provisional explanations of signs or precedents for the purpose of effective intervention, that is, persuasion or healing (98).

Does this insight into the instrumentality of *techne* empty McKeon's architectonic rhetoric of its epistemological implications? No, not entirely. Any product of *techne* is a product that has been made, and so it can be unmade. In this sense, there is a clear connection between *techne* and constructivism, and I see no compelling way of (or reason for) denying it. It goes as far back as Aristotle, who argued that the products of *techne*, unlike those of nature or necessity, have their origin or first principle in a maker, meaning that they depend on human forces to come into being. Yet, despite this dependence, it seems to me that it would be a mistake to assume that by understanding those forces, we also understand the products that they have helped to create. In other words, if the value and significance of *techne*'s products lie in how they are used, not in the products themselves, then getting close to them is not as much a matter of asking how they were made as it is one of asking how they have been made to perform or, even better, how we can make them perform. Here it might be helpful to think back to John Law's argument about how the metaphors of construction and enactment have played out in STS scholarship, an argument

I briefly reviewed at the beginning of chapter 3. According to Law, the first wave of ANT scholarship was dominated by the metaphor of construction, which focused critical attention on science labs and the various inscriptions they produce. Within this paradigm, the goal was to show how these inscriptions, which appeared to be natural and objective facts, were actually constructed by the various inscription devices of the lab.[6] But with the shift to enactment, the goal changed. Attentive to the fact that all sorts of practices beyond the lab participate in the production of reality, and that they do so in order to intervene—"to make a difference in a body or a life"—rather than to describe or tell, scholars began to think about reality not in terms of how (or *that*) objects are brought into existence but rather in terms of how they are performed in practices beyond the scene of their making. Both of these orientations can foster critical engagement, but the second one does not do so on the basis of the reality/appearance distinction that drives constructivist critique. The same, I believe, is true of *techne*, which, as Atwill's commentary highlights, has never been thought of in our field as a kind of inscription device, that is, as a way of producing representational knowledge. Yet this is what is implied by the kind of critique that seeks to show how genetic risk has been rhetorically constructed in ways that make it seem real when it isn't. Can such critique be performed on the products of a *techne* like rhetoric? Yes, but in some sense, it's a mismatch, an exercise in analysis that might not be telling us as much as we think it is. So, to go back to the point I began with—no, this insight into the instrumentality of *techne* does not completely empty McKeon's architectonic productive rhetoric of its epistemological implications. But I would argue that by calling attention to the difference between a kind of production aimed at doing and one aimed at knowing, it does help to mitigate them.

This distinction, or rather, a theoretically complex version of it, gets a more recent treatment in John Muckelbauer's 2008 *The Future of Invention: Rhetoric, Postmodernism, and the Problem of Change*. The eponymous problem to which Muckelbauer responds in this book can be introduced, if not entirely explained, by the clichéd saying that the more things change, the more they stay the same. More accurately, the problem at issue for Muckelbauer is the fact that all of our efforts to achieve difference (that is, to invent) are produced in the same way, through the negative movement of dialectic. No matter what we're after, Muckelbauer argues, difference emerges only by "overcoming or negating particular others—outdated concepts, oppressive social structures, limited subjectivities, or simply undesirable propositions" (4). However, because rejecting this negative movement would entrench rather than solve the problem, Muckelbauer maintains that the future of rhetorical invention depends on our ability to repeat the movement of dialectic more affirmatively, orienting toward the "extraction of singular rhythms" rather than the "extraction of constants" (44).

This distinction between the extraction of singular rhythms and the extraction of constants is what I referred to above as a more theoretically complex version of the distinction between production aimed at doing and production aimed at knowing, and so I want to spend some time here explaining what it means to Muckelbauer and why I've made this comparison. To summarize, the extraction of constants is the standard modus operandi of scholarly engagement, no matter what theoretical position that engagement emanates from. Muckelbauer illustrates this through the examples of humanism and postmodernism, theoretical positions that we would expect to promote very different forms of change. This isn't the case, though, because their modes of engagement or forms of "ethical movement" are exactly the same: they both participate in the negative movement of dialectic by turning the other into a kind of content, that is, something that can be known, critiqued, and replaced (29). The issue here, then, is not about *what* these theoretical positions produce, that is, various arguments about things like subjectivity, agency, language, culture, politics, ethics, and so on. The issue, rather, is *how* they produce it (31–32). In their encounters with each other, both humanism and postmodernism have been inclined toward the extraction of "meanings, things, and contents, *regardless of whether those contents are 'different' or 'the same,' 'new' or 'traditional'*" (35; emphasis added). Thus, they both participate in a "more familiar version of change as negation," one that "seamlessly reintegrates itself into the dialectical movement of appropriation" (35).

Importantly, Muckelbauer argues that in its move from a managerial to an epistemic function, invention came to operate in precisely this way, participating in this same version of change and thus diminishing its actual capacity to create difference.[7] To illustrate, he turns back to *The Prospect of Rhetoric*, showing how its efforts to understand invention very broadly as a "productive human thrust into the unknown" implicitly envisioned the movement of invention as "fundamentally appropriative" (29). "[I]f this generative rhetoric is principally concerned with generating propositions (whether as claims, proof, knowledge, or truth)," Muckelbauer explained, "then this *productive* thrust *into* the unknown would actually function more as a *reproductive* effort to bring something back *from* it, to master the unknown by transforming it into knowledge. Regardless of whether that human thrust is rhetorical (situated) or scientific (objective), the primary axis for its encounters with the unknown is through an effort to change the unknown into knowledge" (29).

So, if this negative movement of dialectic, a movement that Muckelbauer characterizes as the extraction of constants, is the problem, then what is the solution? Or more to the point, what is the solution when any rejection of the negative movement of dialectic would only repeat and entrench that movement? This is the real problem at the heart of Muckelbauer's inquiry into invention, and it is by no means an easy one to solve. If Muckelbauer simply declared that negation was bad, and that we should therefore develop some other mode of scholarly engagement, then he would be participating in the very same kind of change associated with negation. His argument, then, is that we have to repeat the negative movement of dialectic—*but with a difference*. In essence, this is what Muckelbauer means by the extraction of singular rhythms. If we are trapped within the repetitive ethical movement of dialectic, he explains, then "there are innumerable ways of being trapped," that is, "countless different repetitive rhythms" that are "immanent to the actions of identification and signification" yet "manage to go elsewhere" (33). Thus, the difference between the movement of negation and a more affirmative form of invention is one of what Muckelbauer describes as the "inclination" or "pragmatic character" of our response to the other (35). Extracting singular rhythms means being inclined toward the other not "in terms of *what or who the other is*" but rather in terms of the "constellation of forces" that make up any particular "who" or "what" (35). And what such an inclination produces is a kind of "performative mapping" that tries to figure out what a concept can do or what it "can become capable of by connecting it elsewhere" (43).

At one point, Muckelbauer acknowledges that the "rarified terminology" of "extracting singular rhythms" makes his explanation of this more affirmative sense of invention seem exotic when it's not. I think he's right. For that reason, we might turn back to the explanation he offered nine years earlier in "On Reading Differently: Foucault's Resistance," where the styles of engagement under discussion were "productive reading" and "programmatic reading." Programmatic reading corresponds to the extraction of constants insofar as it is an "interpretive attempt to get behind the text, to figure out what an artifact means" (91, 93). Accuracy and representation are key here, and they produce the type of reading that we would associate with a "certain hermeneutic history" of trying to distinguish appearance from reality (91). Within this type of reading, invention is at work, but it is invention as a means to an end, usually the end of making an argument about what's lacking in a particular text. Productive reading, on the other hand, corresponds to the extraction of singular rhythms insofar as its aim is to do something new with the text, to act as a provocation so that "even the most conspicuous lack may mutate into a productive connection" (93). In this style of engagement, Muckelbauer writes, "one reads in order to produce different ideas, to develop possible solutions to contemporary problems, or, as importantly, to move through contemporary problems in an attempt to develop new questions" (74). As in the case of programmatic reading, invention is at work here but not invention as a means to an end or as "one part (or even several parts) of argument formation" (92). Instead, invention itself is the goal, "invention of both concepts and subjects," as one attempts not only to "alter the question, but to alter oneself through the question, to encounter a text hoping to think differently through an engagement with it" (92).

By identifying a style of reading or scholarly engagement in which invention itself is the goal, Muckelbauer has, in some sense, brought us back to McKeon's notion of rhetoric as an architectonic productive art. But this version of the art is not one that we could easily classify as epistemic. Muckelbauer goes to great lengths to explain that the goal of this type of invention is not to better know the other (often by identifying why it's wrong or where it's lacking) but rather to better use the other (or an engagement with it) as a provocation for doing something different.[8] As I argued via my diversion into the meaning of *techne* and its relationship to the metaphor of enactment, I think this distinction between a kind of engagement aimed at knowing and one aimed at doing is actually present in McKeon's version of the art, albeit in a latent way that would not have been useful (or even legible) at a time when rhetoric's disciplinary prospects were so closely yoked to invention's epistemological capacity. But if we take that latent distinction into account, then I think there's a good case for saying that what McKeon means by "perceiving creatively" and what Muckelbauer means by "reading productively" (or extracting singular rhythms) are similar—and not just that they are similar, but also that they exemplify the version of invention that I need in this project, one that does not easily lend itself to constructivist critique and that can therefore justify my effort to develop rhetorical topoi as a way of changing what is happening in this "substantive field" rather than just explaining it.

Of course, Muckelbauer's careful account of the impossibility of doing one of these things without doing the other complicates this effort, but, truthfully, I am grateful for that account since it gives me the language I need for acknowledging what must already be clear from the way that I characterize constructivist critiques of genetic risk throughout this book: the fact that I have engaged in a good deal of programmatic reading and, further, that this won't change as we move into the second half of this chapter. There, I will continue to characterize constructivist critiques of choice and BRCA risk, identifying where I think they go wrong or what I think they are lacking. To the degree that I do this, I have not fully taken up the call issued by Muckelbauer. All I can do here is recognize this inconsistency, pointing out where I do try to take up his call, namely in my engagement with the rhetorics of choice surrounding BRCA risk. My goal here is to read those rhetorics productively (or perceive them creatively) as a way of building something new, in this case, new topoi for thinking, talking, and arguing about the experience of being at genetic risk for breast and ovarian cancers. What makes my encounter with these rhetorics productive, I would argue, is my willingness to acknowledge where they are lacking (a willingness displayed in chapter 1) but then to ask *What can we do with them? Where in these rhetorics is there a potential starting place for a rhetoric of care?* Even this effort is not pure, though. There are moments when my engagement with these rhetorics tilts more toward a diagnosis of their "performative movement" than the production of something new, but my hope is that despite these moments, the net effect of this effort will still be one of invention, not invention solely (or even primarily) as an act of producing content for an argument but also as one of producing tools for making new arguments.

Before moving on to these topics, though, I want to point out that we have come full circle here, which is to say we have returned to Mol's mode of engagement in *The Logic of Care*. While Mol positions her work at the intersection of philosophy and the social sciences, I believe that we can also understand it as an act of rhetorical invention in the sense that I (through the work of McKeon, Atwill, and Muckelbauer) have articulated here. As I explained in chapter 1, Mol's approach to creating a logic of care was primarily ethnographic, meaning that she observed practices and interviewed patients at a diabetes outpatient clinic, collecting a great deal of material about the care that went on there. But her goal was not to explain this material or to use it as a way of explaining reality. To put it in Muckelbauer's terms, she was not trying to extract a content. Rather, she wanted to use her engagement with her material as a way of creating something new—in this case, a language—that could be used to intervene into reality, not just describe or evaluate it. Orienting toward intervention (and invention) in this way does not mean, of course, that the language Mol created *doesn't* correspond to reality or that the events through which she illustrates that language didn't (or don't) happen, only that they aren't common or commonly recognized, and so in order to name them she had to "perceive creatively" or "read productively." As she explains it in the introductory chapter of *The Logic of Care*:

> An anthropologist or sociologist would have taken all of this material and tried to present reality (or part of it) as accurately or as grippingly as possible. However, my aim here is different. I do not seek to sketch a faithful image of the events that I or my informants witnessed. Neither do I want to talk about the meanings of these events for those involved in them. Instead of following the interpretations of my informants, I want to add an interpretation of my own. Instead of relating the perspectives of others, I seek to offer a new perspective. Thus, I have worked with my materials in the way an artist works with paint or with tissue and thread. Or maybe another metaphor is more to the point: I have treated my materials in the way chemists do when faced with a mixed liquid. They distill it to separate out the various components. In a similar way, I have separated out 'good care' from messy practices. In real life, good care co-exists with other logics as well as with neglect and errors. Here I have left out such noise in order to distill a 'pure' form out of mixed events. (10)

As a way *of* moving on to these topics, however, I also want to point out that the language Mol sought to create was a language for describing a *logic*. She wanted to "make words for, and out of, practices" so that we have a way of talking and thinking about the rationales embedded in care practices, ones that have been hard to notice or describe because of the logic of choice (8). What I am after, in contrast, is a set of topics that can help foster a rhetoric of care. To be sure, there is some overlap between my goal and Mol's. The terms she uses to articulate her logic of care look and, as I will show below, can act like topics. But as we've come to know over centuries of trying to define the topics, they can't be understood only in terms of an underlying logic. On the one hand, topics refer to something broader and more flexible than an underlying logic, for instance, lines or patterns of thought (Miller and Selzer 311); indexes of accepted ways of thinking and arguing (Prelli 216); schema for interrelating texts, objects, and writers (Walsh 120); or shared strategies for ordering and investigating experience (Walsh 125). But on the other hand, topics also refer to something different than logic. Over the course of what Muckelbauer describes as their "indescribably diverse and complicated history" (*The Future of Invention* 124) topics have, for example, been understood as indexes of beliefs, values, and attitudes shared by the audience (Leff, "Topics" 23); ways of manifesting ethos (Fahnestock and Secor 91); "bioregions of discourse" (Eberly 6); "aspects of the subject matter under consideration" (Leff 205); "site[s] around which to gather our talk" (Rice 84); regions of "productive uncertainty" that suggest a "conceptual shape" without "specifying its exact contents or connections" (Miller 141); and "ambivalent 'machines' of rhetorical invention that may take verbal or visual expression" (Walsh and Prelli 199).

There is quite a lot of variety in even this brief list of definitions, and if my aim here were to explain once and for all what topoi are, then this variety would be a problem. But in light of what I want these topics to do (help foster a rhetoric of care), the range of definitions and functions is an asset, something I want to capitalize on, not dispel. To return to a point I first made in chapter 1, one of the features that distinguishes my efforts in this book from Mol's efforts in *The Logic of Care* is that they are aimed not only at choice and its limitations within a specific health-care context but also at the constructivist critiques of choice that have dominated our thinking about genetic risk for decades. The rhetoric of care that I hope to foster, in other words, is meant to be an intervention into a broader problem than the one Mol addresses. Thus, it makes sense to aim for a rhetoric (rather than just a logic) of care and to try to build that rhetoric through topoi, which can function in so many different ways. Being able to manifest a different kind of scholarly ethos, for example, is just as important in this effort as being able to identify alternative rationales or warrants for arguments. Here we can see why, as I explained in the introduction, I am indebted not just to Mol's understanding of the term *care* but also to Latour's. In other words, I want these topics to help spur not just a shift from choice to care but also one from engaging BRCA risk as a matter of fact to engaging it as a matter of concern. In some cases, I make this dual purpose explicit, pointing out how I understand the relationship between a topic and these two senses of care, and in others the connections are left implicit. In all cases, though, I begin my discussion of each topic by explaining how I see it functioning within the biosocial discourses of BRCA+ women, and then from there I work out how it could help to foster a rhetoric of care. At times this is more a task of illustration, that is, of actually using the topic, and at others it is more a task of suggesting how it might be used. As readers will quickly realize, while all of these topics traffic in and promote these two senses of care, they don't do so in absolutely distinct ways but instead overlap with one another in an effort to move us away from the well-worn places associated with choice.

Topics of Care

Process, Not Product

I want to begin with this topic, process, not product, for two reasons. First, I have used it before in my own attempts to engage productively with the biosocial discourses surrounding BRCA risk.[9] And second, it is an element of Mol's logic of care and thus provides a transition from her project to mine. As I noted in chapter 1, Mol ends *The Logic of Care* by challenging readers not to passively absorb her book but instead to actively use it. Moving into the health-care contexts relevant to them, she wants readers to think about which elements of her logic of care fit and which don't, which seem worth holding on to and which might be let go (90–91). When I asked myself those questions about this health-care context, I concluded that while almost every element of Mol's logic of care was relevant enough to hold on to, one in particular seemed worth importing into this set of topics, albeit in a revised fashion—process, not product. Perhaps my response had something to do with familiarity. At one point in the history of composition studies, the phrase "process, not product" exceeded the status of disciplinary commonplace to become a rallying cry. Like most rallying cries, it served an important purpose but didn't stand the test of time. Yes, we still find it valuable to distinguish between process-oriented and product-oriented approaches to writing, but few composition scholars would hold up process theory as a sufficient explanation of how writing happens. Within the context of health care, though, process does have something to offer, especially when compared to the competing notion of product in the market version of choice. Recall from chapter 1 Mol's argument that when patients become customers who choose, it only stands to reason that they must have something to choose, and so health care naturally becomes a product, often a "well-delineated product" (20). But in her view, health care should be thought of as a process, one that has no clear boundaries, is open-ended, and will go on for as long as the patient is alive (20).

Clinical Risk Assessments as Informative Facts

It can be hard to think of care in the context of BRCA risk in these terms of process, not product. What genetic medicine provides BRCA+ women is a product, an informative fact, as Mol would call it. This informative fact comes in the form of a clinical risk assessment that indicates if a BRCA mutation was found and, if so, the estimated lifetime risk of cancer that mutation confers. Then, on the basis of this product, BRCA+ women are expected to choose another product, either risk-reducing surgery or high-risk cancer surveillance. They have become BRCA+ by virtue of this informative fact, and everything, every decision and every step going forward, will follow from it.

This product-oriented approach to BRCA risk and the rhetoric of choice it fosters is easy to spot in the FORCE message boards, where women often begin posts about their health-care choices by saying that they *are* BRCA1 or BRCA2. We can also see this approach in the broader biosocial literature, especially BRCA guidebooks, which, in some cases, are organized in terms of a pre- and post-testing chronology. *Confronting Hereditary Breast and Ovarian Cancer*, for instance, transitions readers from part 2 of the book, "Assessing Your Risk," to part 3, "Managing Your Risk," with a section called "Now What? Implications for You and Your Family." There readers are counseled to remember that everyone reacts differently to a positive BRCA result, but whatever a woman's reaction, she must now make "some difficult decisions" about managing her risk (Friedman 71). The transition in *Previvors* is similar, if somewhat more forceful, as it warns readers that once they know they have a good chance of developing breast or ovarian cancer, they have two choices: either they "do nothing" and hope to "beat the odds," or they "take action" and try to "defy [. . . their] fate" (Port 57). It would seem that doing nothing is not a real option, as the very next sentence advises readers to "rely on a team of experts such as surgeons, oncologists, gynecologists, genetics experts, and psychologists" to figure out what to do next (57).

Critics have long pointed out the problems with this product-oriented approach, even if they haven't identified it in those terms. In fact, we might argue that critiques of geneticization are, in essence, critiques of this approach. To claim that an illness or condition has been geneticized, as, for instance, Hoedemaekers and Ten Have did in their study of beta thalassemia or Margaret Lock did in her study of breast cancer, is to claim that on account of one piece of information, what Lock calls the "decontextualized findings of basic science," patients identify as at risk and engage in whatever preventative measures are deemed necessary to protect their health (13). As we saw in chapter 3, Happe made a similar claim about ovarian cancer, arguing that clinical risk assessments operate as a "distinct epistemological category" that provides an "indisputable basis for action" and devalues the more situated, material, and lived form of knowledge about genetic risk that mutation carriers get from family history (79–80). In other words, the "putatively real risk" associated with clinical risk assessments makes BRCA+ women "unqualified candidates" for prophylactic bilateral salpingo-oophorectomy, with the only exception being those who want children and are young enough to have them (90, 93). Thus, it is by obtaining the one product, the informative fact of the clinical risk assessment, that BRCA+ women are put on a very narrow path toward choosing another product, risk-reducing surgery.

Although I understand the rationale behind arguments like Happe's, I worry that by critiquing this product-oriented approach, we only reinforce it and, worse, that it keeps us from recognizing or offering any kind of alternative. Taking a cue from Mol, then, I want to ask what the idea of process might offer us in this specific medical context. If product is a common topic in the discourses surrounding BRCA risk, serving as an index of an accepted way of thinking for both those who advocate it and those who critique it, then what could process offer as an alternative? Can it also become an index of an accepted way of thinking, and if so, what would that entail? What would it allow us to see differently? How might it help foster a rhetoric of care?

To begin answering these questions, I want to turn back to Mol's notion of informative facts. It's here, in the possibility of rethinking this element of the logic and the rhetorics of choice, that I think process can make a contribution to a rhetoric of care. As I explained in chapter 1, Mol argues that among the traits shared by both versions of the logic of choice is a tendency to treat scientific knowledge as a collection of informative facts that doctors disseminate to patients, who, once in possession of the facts, add in values and make a choice (*Logic of Care* 42–43). Mol's problem with this feature of the logic of choice is that it elides the messiness of medicine, that is, the fact that facts and values are intertwined and, further, that what counts as a medical or scientific fact cannot be determined outside the context of care practices and patients' lives (45–46). Thus, she proposes target values as an alternative, arguing that in the logic of care, facts do not precede decisions about how to intervene. Target values are what doctors aim for, and they do this during treatment, not before it (46).

Although Mol doesn't talk about informative facts and target values in relation to product- and process-oriented approaches to health care, it's easy to see
how the two former terms are a subset of the latter two. Informative facts correspond to a product-oriented approach to health care insofar as they are pieces
of information that allow doctors and patients to act, while target values correspond to a process-oriented approach insofar as they are something that
doctors and patients must determine *as* they act. As I have already noted, the
idea of informative facts works well as a description of the product that genetic
medicine offers BRCA+ women, namely a clinical risk assessment. But Mol's
notion of target values doesn't work as well as an alternative in the context of
BRCA risk as it does in that of diabetes, where doctors and patients are continually trying to determine what blood sugar levels will provide optimal health.
And so in order to demonstrate what process can offer us as a rhetorical topic, I
want to use it as a way to rethink the nature and function of clinical risk assessments. That is, I want to ask how we might see this particular kind of informative fact differently if we assume, despite what the rhetorics of choice tell us, that
care in the context of BRCA risk is a process that has no clear boundaries, is
open-ended, and will go on for as long as the patient is alive.

Clinical Risk Assessments as Interpretable Signs

To be fair, if we were to make this assumption about care in the context of
BRCA risk, then we would not be the first. Although the biosocial discourses
surrounding BRCA risk are overwhelmingly product-oriented, especially in
terms of how they regard the nature and value of a clinical risk assessment, there
are moments when a more process-oriented approach comes into view. Take, for
example, the very last paragraph of *Confronting Hereditary Breast and Ovarian
Cancer*, the BRCA guidebook co-authored by FORCE founder Sue Friedman.
It's worth noting that this paragraph immediately follows the two decision-
making guides that I described in chapter 1, "Comparing Risk-Reducing Alternatives" and "From Confused to Clear in Fifteen Steps."

> Hereditary cancer doesn't end with a decision. Each answer, test result,
> and choice means sacrifice, and every sacrifice requires adjustment. You
> move forward step by step; each one requires emotional investment, usu-
> ally followed with a period of grieving, accepting uncertainty, and adjust-
> ing to changes. No matter which course of action you choose, you must
> live with the consequences, whether or not things go according to plan. At

some point, moving forward becomes a leap of faith that you've gathered as much information as you need, you know what to expect from the actions you decide upon, and you've chosen the best path forward. If the unexpected occurs—as it sometimes does—be patient and forgiving with yourself, and know that you made the best decision that you could at the time. Then move on to the next set of decisions and deal with what lies ahead. In this way, we move forward and eventually allow ourselves to find joy in life and live it to the fullest. (236)

If care is to be understood in Mol's terms as what patients do to live a good life when what they want (perfect health) is out of reach, then I would say that in this paragraph we find a trenchant example of a rhetoric of care, one that stems from and promotes a process-oriented approach to living with BRCA risk. Yet it doesn't tell us much about clinical risk assessments, about how such a process-oriented approach might allow us to see them as something other than informative facts. For that, I want to turn to the FORCE message boards, looking at one of the ways clinical risk assessments function when BRCA+ women have to make the difficult choice between surgery and surveillance. What makes this decision between surgery and surveillance so hard is that there are two kinds of cancer to think about and, further, the fact that both of them affect the bodily features and capacities most obviously associated with womanhood. Thus, as we might imagine, some BRCA+ women are reluctant to choose risk-reducing surgery as their means of managing both breast and ovarian cancer risk, since the prospect of having both one's breasts and one's ovaries removed not only carries the risk of severe iatrogenic side effects but also poses too drastic a threat to identity. In some instances, then, the specific decision-making dilemma is one of determining which surgery at which time will be the most beneficial—bilateral mastectomy or bilateral salpingo-oophorectomy?

Clinical risk assessments obviously play an important role in this decision-making situation, and it's easy to identify instances where they function rhetorically as an informative fact, that is, as an "indisputable basis for action," as Happe puts it. But there are also times when, working in tandem with familial risk assessments, or family history, they don't wield quite so much authority. The fact that BRCA+ women combine these two kinds of information about risk is hardly a surprising observation. Naturally, they would want to marshal as much evidence as possible when making and justifying such high-stakes health-care decisions. But the relationship between clinical and familial risk assessments is not always simply additive or supplemental. Rather, the familial risk assessment can work as a lens for unlocking or deciphering the information perceived to be embedded in the clinical risk assessment, making the latter more of an interpretable sign than an informative fact.

A sign, of course, is something that stands for something else, or, as Charles Sanders Pierce put it, it is "something which by knowing we know something more" (quoted in Johansen and Larson 25). But what, in the case of a clinical risk assessment, is this "something more"? That is, what do BRCA+ women know by virtue of this sign? On the one hand, we can say that they know they inherited a mutated BRCA1 or BRCA2 gene. From this point of view, I have to admit, it actually does make sense to think of a clinical risk assessment as an informative fact—something that is determined outside the context of care practices and patients' lives. Or, to stick with Pierce's terminology, we could say that as signs, clinical risk assessments function in the indexical mode, meaning they indicate a "genuine relation" between the sign and the object it stands for. In this case, that relation is one of inheritance. Clinical risk assessments indicate that a mutation in either the BRCA1 or BRCA2 gene was passed down from a parent to a child in an autosomal dominant fashion. This event of "passing down" happened, and the object to which the sign refers is "necessarily existent," operating in some sense as a constraint on that sign (Chandler 37). Of course, this is not the same kind of indexical relation that exists between a sign like smoke and an object like fire, where the former is actually modified by the latter, but it also doesn't rely on the "interpreting mind" in the way that another kind of sign in Pierce's taxonomy, symbolic signs, do.

Symbolic signs, as we know, are not modified by the objects they stand for; rather, their relationship is either arbitrary or conventional, and so we do have to rely on the "interpreting mind" in order to know what that "something more" is. Because BRCA mutations do not have 100 percent penetrance, meaning that no one can predict how or if they will affect the health of a carrier, clinical risk assessments also function in this mode, requiring BRCA+ women to engage in an interpretive process in order to figure out what they mean. As I noted earlier, familial risk assessments can play a key role in this process, acting as a lens for deciphering that meaning. Take, for example, the following post from a FORCE message board thread started by a BRCA+ woman who had decided on bilateral salpingo-oophorectomy but was conflicted about bilateral mastectomy. In her initial post, this woman explained that although her sister died from breast cancer and she herself has an "87% chance" of developing the disease, she cannot proceed with PBM. Feeling "stuck," she asked how others decided on prophylactic surgery. One BRCA+ woman offered the following explanation:

> BSO was easy probably due to my age, 49 y/o. PBM was much harder to "wrap my head around." My husband said it was like killing a gnat with an elephant gun. It took me two years to decide on PBM. During those two years, I learned as much as I could about procedures, results, risks, etc. Then my cousin who was diagnosed with Stage I breast cancer at 32 relapsed at 40. She had two young children. This was my ah ha moment. It was also the point that my husband came to terms with the seriousness of my BRCA status. This is when I went through with the PBM.

Here, we can see a key reason why familial risk assessments can function as an interpretive lens for clinical risk assessments: they can incorporate several kinds of risk information, for example, not only information about chances of developing disease but also information about chances of detecting, treating, and surviving it. For these BRCA+ women, such information is crucial, as mainstream breast cancer culture is known for its intense focus on the link between early detection, successful treatment, and survival. For nearly forty years, messages to get surveilled and to surveil oneself have been promulgated on the premise that breast cancer is survivable when caught early. Predictably, then, within this cultural context, an event such as the relapse of a cousin's Stage I breast cancer eight years after diagnosis could refine a clinical risk assessment, suggesting, for instance, that one's actual lifetime risk is at the upper end of the spectrum or that one is at risk of a particularly aggressive type of breast cancer.

To be clear, though, the result of this interpretive process is not always a feeling of cancer's "inevitability" and thus a choice to have surgery. To the contrary, as family histories and personal experiences of disease differ, so do the interpretations and decisions that BRCA+ women come to. Take, for instance, the following post from a different FORCE message board thread started by another woman who had no reservations about PBSO but was not ready for PBM. Leaning toward surveillance, she asked others for input. A BRCA1 mutation carrier responded, explaining that she chose surveillance for her breasts and surgery for her ovaries. Asked if her decision-making process was easy, she wrote:

The ooph was an easy decision for me, a no-brainer. My mother's ovca was Stage 3B when it was found. She was in the best shape of her life, running long distance, lifting weights. She had no idea she had cancer. Her survival chances were slim and it was amazing that she survived. Knowing that, the decision to do the ooph was easy. [. . .] There was a study on FORCE that really drives home the benefit of doing the ooph. If I'm remembering correctly, doing nothing gave you a 50% chance of making it to 70. Doing the ooph gave you an 80% chance of making it to 70. And doing the ooph + PBM gave you an 84% chance of making it to 70. So for me it became a quality of life decision. Do I want to skip the PBM surgery and quite possibly have to go through breast cancer, or do I want to undergo major surgery, give up my breasts, and most likely not have to go through breast cancer? I came down on the surveillance side of the fence, but certainly understand why other people come down on the PBM side of the fence. There's no guarantee that I would follow in my mother's footsteps, but her bc was caught early and treated easily. AND since people didn't know about BRCA back then, she fell into the "do nothing" category and DID make it to 70. That gives me huge hope.

As a BRCA1 mutation carrier, this woman has an approximately 50 percent to 80 percent lifetime chance of developing breast cancer and a 24 percent to 40 percent lifetime chance of developing ovarian cancer (Petrucelli). Yet read through family history, this clinical risk assessment acquires a more specific meaning, referring not only to her chances of getting these diseases but also to her chances of detecting, treating, and surviving them. Thus, by making this shift from informative fact to interpretable sign (or, more broadly, from product to process), we might argue that while clinical risk assessments are absolutely taken to be real by BCRA+ women like the above message board contributor, they are not regarded as unified or indisputable. In other words, we might argue that already at work in the biosocial discourses of some BRCA+ women is a recognition that the interpretability of clinical risk assessments does not diminish their reality but rather adds to it by drawing in familial risk assessments and making them an important part of the decision-making process. Rather than devaluing this older, more situated form of knowledge about genetic risk, then, clinical risk assessments and the decision-making situations they necessitate could be said to repurpose or reprioritize familial risk assessment, demonstrating that for BRCA+ women, making decisions about health care is not a zero-sum game where to accede reality to one kind of information about risk is to subtract it from the other.

Process as Means of Disentangling Good Care from Good Choices

If the goal is to foster a rhetoric of care, then the value of an argument like this one is fairly self-evident. It focuses our attention on Mol's notion of care insofar as it gives us a way of thinking about clinical risk assessments as something other than well-delineated products, and it brings in Latour's understanding of the term insofar as it allows us to see that for some BRCA+ women, the reality of those risk assessments is not diminished by their need to be interpreted in the light of familial risk assessments. But the potential of this topic is not limited to this example argument about clinical risk assessments. Arguably, its impact could be much broader, as it could offer us a rhetorical mechanism for distinguishing between what counts as a good choice and what counts as good care in the context of BRCA risk. As I noted in chapter 1, we often think of the BRCA experience in terms of "bifurcation points" like testing versus not testing or having surgery versus undergoing surveillance. While it makes sense to think in these terms (since there are, in fact, many irreversible choices BRCA+ women must make), I would argue that they have helped to collapse the distinction between care and choice, encouraging us to define the former in terms of the latter. The rhetorical topic of process could help diminish this confusion by grounding our thinking in a set of assumptions (e.g., that care has no clear boundaries, is open-ended, and will go on for as long as the patient is alive) that force us to take a longer view of BRCA risk, looking past the initial point of decision making to the everyday medical interactions and practices that are part of life for those at genetic risk of breast and ovarian cancers.

Quality of Life

This second topic, quality of life, is a prominent part of the rhetoric of choice surrounding BRCA risk, showing up often in the FORCE message boards, as well as in several of the interviews I conducted. Hannah, for instance, couched her decision to have PBM in these terms, explaining that for her, quality of life is "huge," and that she's often frustrated by how people "downplay" its importance when they talk about the pros and cons of prophylactic surgery. Carrie made a similar argument about PBSO, explaining that every time she "had a little cramp," she was "freaked out," and that she eventually came to feel that "this is not a way to live." After describing how "tough" her PBM surgery was, a FORCE message board contributor declared that she would "do it a hundred times over for this new quality of life it has brought." Another wrote that after "millions" of doctor appointments and "tons of lost sleep," she realized her "quality of life was uber sucking," as she "failed to negotiate the fear and stress with grace." "I wanted my life back," she explained, even if that meant trading natural breasts for reconstructed ones. In each of these examples, we see quality of life being used as a way to justify the choice to have prophylactic surgery, with the implication being that surveillance is too much to bear. But in keeping with the notion of topoi as tools for arguing both sides of an issue, this topic functions just as well for those who've decided not to have surgery, especially PBSO since its side effects can so drastically diminish quality of life. In a FORCE message board thread about having oophorectomy with or without hysterectomy, for instance, a women with a BRCA1 mutation explained that even though she knew she wasn't going to have children, she couldn't proceed with PBSO because she was "terrified" about what it might do her quality of life. In *Blood Matters*, Masha Gessen framed her decision not to have PBSO in similar terms, writing that even though she was well aware of studies showing increased life expectancy for women who had the surgery, she couldn't get past the idea that this increase was "an absurdly small gain in exchange for drastically lowering [her] quality of life" (83). Ultimately, she decided to have a PBM but avoid the PBSO and live with the 40 percent lifetime ovarian cancer risk conferred by her BRCA1 mutation.

Quality of Life and Values Beyond Autonomy

These examples demonstrate that within the rhetoric of choice, quality of life is a useful topic for women at genetic risk of breast and ovarian cancers. It does important rhetorical work for them as they carry out their role as health-care citizens, deliberating about which paths are best in light of their personal preferences and circumstances. But what kind of work can it do within a rhetoric of care? Or, more accurately, what can it do to help foster a rhetoric of care? To answer this question, it's helpful to consider Carolyn Miller's argument about the topics and venatic thinking in "The Aristotelian *Topos*: Hunting for Novelty," an argument that I briefly mentioned earlier. If, as she argues there, topics function by locating us within "a region of general conception," then to understand how this topic could foster a rhetoric of care, we might ask what, in the case of quality of life, is in that region (141)? In other words, what comes with the territory here? What's already part of the conversation, even if we are not arguing *about* quality of life per se? Perhaps most obviously (and somewhat like the first topic), quality of life evokes images of medical problems that cannot be easily or immediately cured, but whose effects can be mitigated or managed through treatment. Treatment, however, often brings its own set of problems (e.g., side effects, loss of effectiveness over time, inconvenience, and financial burden), and so quality of life also evokes notions of compromise, of having to figure out which problems are worth dealing with and which ones aren't. Compromise, in turn, evokes a reality in which patients cannot have everything they want but through some effort and sacrifice can still try to live a good life despite the limitations imposed by illness and/or its treatment. Trying to live a good life despite such limitations is, in fact, a good way to think about quality of life and the broad definition of health it implies. That definition includes people's physical, mental, and emotional functioning in relation to disease status, but it extends beyond that to also incorporate their well-being, life satisfaction, and ability to participate in the world around them ("Health-Related Quality of Life and Well-Being").

As even this short discussion indicates, much of what is "in" the region specified by quality of life overlaps with the notion of care as Mol has defined it. In particular, there is a common emphasis on the imbrication of health care with life and all those aspects of it (work, family, desires, habits, etc.) that can complicate our efforts to achieve and maintain good health. Mol, however, doesn't use the phrase "quality of life" in *The Logic of Care*, and I suspect that choice has something to do with the way that work on this subject pits patient and professional perspectives against one another, often framing the former's subjectivity as the necessary corrective to latter's objectivity.[10] Although this split between subjective and objective realities in medicine is more of a concern for her in *The Body Multiple* than in *The Logic of Choice*, there is still a sensitivity to this problem in the later book, and so despite its connections to care, quality of life is not something Mol talks about. But it is something BRCA+ women talk about, and even if that talk happens mainly within a rhetoric of choice (or maybe *because* it happens within a rhetoric of choice), it can work in subtle ways to highlight the kind of constrained acting that goes on within this particular health-care context. As we saw in chapter 1, within the rhetoric of choice that surrounds BRCA risk, what matters most is the ability to choose freely. But is anyone who thinks, talks, or acts in terms of quality of life really free to choose what she wants? Aren't other values besides autonomy always already at work in situations where quality of life is either an issue or a reasonable way of framing an issue? In making this observation, I am not suggesting that it is our job to argue about or adjudicate among these values, only that choice itself produces rhetorical counter-currents that can help to foster a rhetoric of care.

Quality of Life and the Line Between Health and Disease

If quality of life, as a rhetorical topic, can draw our attention to these other values, then I think it has significant potential for fostering a rhetoric of care. Moreover, it helps us to see what else "fits," as Mol put it, or where there is similarity between these two contexts, diabetes and BRCA risk. But as I've argued throughout this book, when we move into the context of BRCA risk, the problem a rhetoric of care must respond to is not just the rhetoric of choice but also the critiques of choice that have developed in response to that rhetoric. As chapter 2 demonstrated, those critiques have unfolded in a number of ways, but one common move has been for critics to turn to the discourses, narratives, and ideologies surrounding genetic rick, showing how they muddy the line between health and disease, thereby compelling BRCA+ women to engage in medical interventions (e.g., PBM and PBSO) that even further muddy that line. Think, for instance, of Happe's question about how it becomes "thinkable" for BRCA+ women to undergo the same medical treatment as ovarian cancer patients. In chapter 3, I offered an alternative explanation of this kind of overlap between health and disease, arguing that it is a tension in medicine, one that we can explain but not one we can explain away. Here, I offer something related but simpler, namely the observation that this kind of critique depends on a very narrow definition of health as the absence of disease. This definition is not usually made explicit, but if it were, the argument would go like this: if health is the absence of disease, and those who are "simply BRCA positive" do not have disease, then they are healthy, and therefore anything—any intervention, ideology, or narrative—that suggests otherwise is suspect and thus subject to critique. The logic underlying this argument is sound enough, but the suspicion it breeds is antithetical to a rhetoric of care. How can we find ways of engaging BRCA risk as a matter of concern and of thinking of BRCA+ women as patients who act even when they cannot choose if we are working with a definition of health that keeps us poised for purification, always on the look out for the aberration or infringement that has disempowered someone?

What a topic like quality of life can do, then, is diminish the grounds for that suspicion by locating us in a region where health is more than the absence of disease. The definition I cited above does this, as does any other that shifts our focus beyond just disease status to the impact of health care on patients' lives. To appreciate the significance of this impact, we need only think back to the women whose experiences of breast cancer screening I described in chapter 3, women whose bodies were enacted as uncertain sources of knowledge about cancer, even (or especially) when testing produced no evidence of disease. Indeed, these women did not have cancer, and on this basis we could say they were healthy. But could we say they were receiving good care? Or, more to the point, could we say that we were helping them receive good care, that our typical ways of talking and arguing about BRCA risk were capable of such a thing?

If BRCA risk is the kind of messy object I described in chapter 3, then we must consider the possibility that the answer to this last question is often *no* and that, in fact, efforts to maintain the distinction between health and disease can impede our ability to advocate for good care for BRCA+ women. Built from the topic of quality of life, then, a chief goal of a rhetoric of care would be to normalize this blurring between health and disease so that we might find new ways of talking about care for BRCA+ women. What happens, for instance, if we talk about cancer screening as medical treatment for a chronic condition? In other words, what happens if we rhetorically acknowledge this reality of BRCA risk, the fact by virtue of *some* practices, it can be enacted as a chronic condition? Wouldn't this shift make it easier to ask how those practices can be administered with more care? Wouldn't it help us better account for the cumulative effects of screening on the at-risk body? And wouldn't it, in this sense, help us to see that it is this body, not just a woman's subjective understanding of her cancer risk, that is at stake in this mode of enacting BRCA risk? If so, then I would argue that the potential of this topic lies not just in its ability to diminish the grounds for the suspicion that drives purification but more specifically (and productively) in its ability to enhance the grounds for a fuller consideration of the at-risk body. Defining health as more than the absence of disease makes room for this body. It allows that body to show up as something that matters even though it is not diseased *and* even though it is not in need of emancipation. Saying what this body needs if not emancipation is no easy task. Of course, we can (and should) say that it needs BRCA risk to be a less messy object, one that doesn't overlap so easily with disease through the problem of false positive test results, for instance. But unless or until that change happens, a rhetoric of care can help us say what else the at-risk body needs by acknowledging that messiness and framing it—for physicians, patients, and critics—as part of the reality of BRCA risk.

Between the Devil and the Deep

If there is something "in" the region specified by quality of life that implies BRCA+ women are constrained, unable to choose freely because what they want (to not have a BRCA mutation, for instance) is not possible, then this third topic, being between the devil and the deep, makes that predicament explicit. To be between the devil and the deep is to have no good choices, and while the BRCA+ women who employ this topic don't always do so with the same terminology, the arguments they craft with it have a similar effect insofar as they challenge the rhetoric of choice that tells them they should feel grateful for and empowered by the "strong options" that knowledge of a BRCA mutation brings. In chapter 1, I showed how these messages about gratitude and empowerment are communicated in BRCA guidebooks and high-profile texts like the 2013 op-ed where Jolie used that phrase, "strong options," to describe the medical situation for BRCA+ women, but they are just as common in less "official" types of biosocial discourse. Frequently on the FORCE message boards, contributors express gratitude for the chance to be proactive, and, as we saw in chapter 1, two of the women I interviewed, Gina and Cheri, did as well, telling me that knowledge of their mutations made them feel lucky, empowered, and better prepared than those for whom a cancer diagnosis might come as a surprise.

No Good Choices

For women who feel less optimistic than Gina and Cheri about BRCA risk, it's easy to see why a topic like being between the devil and the deep would be rhetorically useful, especially within the context of a biosocial community like FORCE, which is known for its proactive, positive attitude about BRCA risk. This attitude is reflected in the term *previvor*, which was coined by FORCE message board contributors in 2000 to refer to anyone who is a "survivor of a predisposition to cancer." As Tasha Dubriwny argues in *The Vulnerable Empowered Woman*, the previvor identity is "based fundamentally on an optimistic view of life and science and the belief that once an individual is empowered to make choices, cancer can be conquered or simply avoided altogether" (43). But what if there are no good choices? What if all possible choices are equally bad? If this is that case, then one can reasonably question what there is to be grateful for or empowered by. Moreover, if there are no good choices, then feelings of frustration, despair, disappointment, doubt, anger, or anything contrary to gratitude and empowerment are justified, even natural. What a topic like being between the devil and the deep can do, then, is provide a means of expressing feelings, ideas, and arguments that run counter to the ethos of the community (and arguably the ethos of the new genetics more broadly) while still demonstrating one's membership in it. Take, for example, the following FORCE post by a woman with a BRCA1 mutation who turned to the message boards because she wanted to know if anyone else had considered PBM but then decided against it:

> My story—Am 48. Brca1. Had an ooph at 38. Been on hrt [hormone replacement therapy] ever since, despite which libido is affected. And parts dont [sic] function as well as before. I have made peace with it though. I havent not [sic] however been able to plunge into the pbm even though I have met with some of the best doctors who assure me that they can give me back a bit of sensation and a natural feel after diep [deep inferior epigastric perforator reconstruction]. All my doctors (at Sloan Kett) are in favor of a pbm. I feel them steering me there all the time. My mom is a 26 year ovca survivor. This year at 73 she got an early breast cancer. She refused chemo and hated having a lumpectomy. She would never want either one of us to have a mastectomy unless it was absolutely mandatory. After Angelina Jolie's disclosure I felt a bit better about it. But that has faded now and I am back to living with my doubts. A pbm seems so brutal and such a fear based decision. The fact that so many women are opting for it is quite an indictment of the cancer establishment who still havent [sic] come up with a cure or reasonable treatments. Does any one know of any new tests coming up? I would like to volunteer for chemo or nano prevention. Meanwhile, I am going with surveillance, which almost killed me last time as I had to have a biopsy—totally terrifying. Talk about being between the devil and the deep.

That this BRCA+ woman has had a hard time deciding between risk-reducing surgery and cancer surveillance does not make her unique. Arguably no dilemma (or bifurcation point) is more central to the BRCA experience than having to make a decision between surgery and surveillance. However, at the heart of her dilemma, at least as it is presented here, is a different problem than the one we normally see in the biosocial discourses surrounding BRCA risk. Within those discourses, the difficulty of deciding between surgery and surveillance is typically framed as the difficulty of figuring out which option better fits a woman's personal preferences and life circumstances. *How much risk can she tolerate? Does she want children, and if so, does she want to breastfeed them? Can she handle the grinding routine of surveillance? What is her family history and how has it impacted her?* Clearly these are hard questions to answer, and they illustrate well why this is such a tough choice for women. But in the FORCE message board post above, making a decision is difficult for a different reason, namely that the choices are both so bad, either a "brutal" surgery or a lifetime of potentially "terrifying" experiences with breast cancer screening. Neither option is acceptable to this BRCA+ woman, and so she turns to the idea of being stuck between the devil and the deep to express her frustration and doubt. Is she using this idea in the same way we might use a topic like definition or opposites, that is, turning to it intentionally in order to support a claim she wants her audience to accept? No, I don't believe that she is. In fact, it is fairly clear here that feeling stuck between two equally undesirable options *is* her claim, not the means by which she is trying to support some other claim. Nevertheless, by framing her frustration and doubt in relation to such a difficult dilemma, this BRCA+ woman legitimizes (or at least rationalizes) those feelings, thereby helping to create a place from which she and other BRCA+ women can challenge the too-easy association of having choices with being empowered.

Both Hannah and Carrie turned to this place when I talked to them about the testing and risk-reducing practices they had participated in; however, they were much more explicit in their rejection of the relationship between choice and empowerment. Carrie, for instance, explained that her friends thought she was brave for having a PBSO at such a young age, but that "no part" of her actually felt that way. She had the surgery because she had just watched her BRCA2+ uncle die of pancreatic cancer, and she thought it was better to "suffer through some miserable surgeries and possibly look dramatically different and maybe not feel great and be all hot-flashy and menopausal" than to live with surveillance and increased ovarian cancer risk. "That's really the thing with BRCA," she explained, "there are a lot of choices, and they're all terrible," and so while some of her BRCA Facebook friends felt very empowered by their ability to choose, Carrie did not. On a good day she felt that something positive had come out of her uncle's death, but for her that wasn't the same thing as empowerment; at most it "was a nice thought every once in a while." Hannah felt similarly, explaining that yes, she had chosen to get tested for a BRCA mutation, and yes, she had chosen to have a PBM, but she had not necessarily made those choices freely. If she had chosen not to test for the BRCA2 mutation in her family, then she knew the doctors would treat her as though she had it, subjecting her to the intense cancer-screening regimen recommended for all BRCA+ women. Thus for her, the decision to test "didn't even feel like a choice." "There was never really any, like, should I or shouldn't I," she told me. If she was going to be able to avoid a lifetime of surveillance, she *had* to test. Her thinking about PBM proceeded along similar lines. She knew that if she didn't have the PBM and was later diagnosed with breast cancer, she would be told she needed not just a mastectomy but most likely chemotherapy as well. So Hannah chose the PBM, reasoning that she'd rather do it on her terms than someone else's. But that didn't mean she thought the surgery was a good choice. Like Carrie, Hannah felt that there were no good choices for BRCA+ women, and, as a result, she was uncomfortable with the word "empowerment" and the way it "gets flung around so easily" when people talk about BRCA risk. "I feel better that I made these choices but I don't feel empowered. I feel a little bit more in control and I feel a little more at peace but it's not as though I'm ready to put on my superwoman costume and go out there and fight cancer. It doesn't feel like that at all."

Constrained but Not Disempowered

Insofar as this topic, being between the devil and the deep, provides BRCA+ women a place from which they can challenge the too-easy association of having choices with being empowered, then I believe it has the potential to foster a rhetoric of care. When women like Carrie and Hannah talk about the medical practices they've participated in in terms of having no good choices, they implicitly acknowledge the importance of values other than autonomy. And when a FORCE message board poster writes about her decision-making process in terms of being stuck between the devil and the deep, she shows how she can be dissatisfied but still part of her proactive biosocial community. What happens, though, when *we* talk and write in these terms? That is, of what value is a topic like being between the devil and the deep not just for BRCA+ women but also for us, critics in the humanities and social sciences? One answer to this question is that by challenging the too-easy association of *not* having choices with being *dis*empowered, this topic could provide a place for developing a feminist perspective on BRCA risk. Of course, there already is a feminist perspective on BRCA risk, one that, as we saw in chapter 2, has produced a significant amount of critical discourse about the social functions of genetic risk. But often that perspective is so colored by the past successes of feminist breast cancer activism that it elides important differences between sporadic and hereditary forms of cancer.[11] Take, for example, Dubriwny's critique of the "PM narrative" in chapter 3 of *The Vulnerable Empowered Woman*. Her central claim is that this narrative has all of the feminist trappings of the women's health movement of the 1970s but none of the substance. That is, through its emphasis on gaining knowledge, taking action, and "bodily self-determination," this narrative promises empowerment but cannot actually deliver on that promise because all of the choices it offers BRCA+ women are compulsory choices that demand not just compliance with heterosexist norms about personal responsibility and female bodies but also an unquestioning consumption of biomedicine (54, 55–58). It is in this sense that Dubriwny sees the PM narrative as an extension of a mainstream breast cancer culture that for decades now has turned breast cancer into a disease of the individual and ignored its environmental and social causes. Indeed, in her view, "[a]dding the science of genetics to the rhetoric of risk surrounding breast cancer" hasn't changed anything, not the "overall message of choice and personal responsibility, not the blindness to issues of race and class (35), and certainly not the close relationship with biomedicine that has left little room for questioning breast cancer research and treatments (151–52). Thus for Dubriwny, what is needed is a genuinely feminist perspective on BRCA risk, one that by allowing BRCA+ women to question medical experts and the treatments they promote can help them find real empowerment.[12]

In the very beginning of *The Logic of Care*, Mol acknowledges how hard it is to question choice. In most arenas in life, having choices is better than not having them, and so we are rightfully suspicious of anyone who argues otherwise. It is similarly hard to question questioning. Common sense tells us it is better to question the treatments offered by the medical-industrial complex than to accept them uncritically, especially in a situation like this, where healthy women are having their breasts and ovaries surgically removed to prevent diseases they might not get. No one wants BRCA+ women to be uncritical consumers of such treatments, and no situation, it would seem, cries out louder for a feminist critique of compulsory choice. Yet I think we have to ask ourselves where such critique leaves BRCA+ women. What, for instance, do we imagine we are offering them when we explain that their choice to have a PBM is the result of a cultural narrative that says women must sacrifice anything (even healthy body parts) in order to be alive to have and raise children? Or when we argue that by having prophylactic surgery, they're mistaking their risk of disease for disease and, through that mistake, becoming "responsibilized" as good neoliberal, postfeminist subjects? What do we expect them to do with this information? Or, more to the point, do we expect that this kind of information will empower them to choose differently? This really is the heart of the matter here—whether or not questioning the lack of choice surrounding BRCA risk empowers BRCA+ women to choose differently. Questioning procedures like the one-step biopsy and the Halstead radical mastectomy in the 1970s was empowering not just because it identified the rampant sexism of biomedicine but also because it helped lead to better care—for instance, two-step procedures that allowed patients to be informed of their diagnoses before surgery and mastectomies that removed the entire breast but not the chest wall muscles. More recently, questioning the necessity of mastectomy for localized sporadic cancers has led to greater use of breast-conserving therapies like lumpectomy. There's not a BRCA+ woman alive who doesn't hope for a similar movement toward less invasive procedures for cancer prevention. We would be remiss, however, if we did not acknowledge that in these past instances of feminist breast cancer activism, the procedures that most clearly embodied the sexism of biomedicine were also the ones that did not provide the best medical care. That they were practiced despite their deficiencies speaks very loudly to the power of that sexism. But what if for BRCA+ women, the procedures that most clearly embody the sexism of biomedicine are also the ones that currently provide the best medical care, even if that care leaves much to be desired? And what if in our attempts to bring a feminist perspective to bear on BRCA risk, we are not only eliding important differences between sporadic and hereditary forms of cancer but also engaging in a form of purification that reduces those procedures to some pretty reprehensible "social stuff"? Where does such a reduction leave BRCA+ women? Peter Sloterdijk would probably argue that it leaves them in the very cynical place of having to knowingly follow an illusion. Latour might say that it leaves them a little bruised, with no rug beneath their feet. To these observations I would simply add (or clarify, since I am making a similar point) that there is a very good chance it does not leave them empowered because as reprehensible as that "social stuff" might be, it neither disqualifies surgery as a reasonable response to BRCA risk nor makes the alternative, a lifetime of cancer screening, a truly good option.

At the heart of this topic, being between the devil and the deep, is the idea that there are *no* truly good choices for BRCA+ women. That is what is "in" this region or normative from this point of view, and a feminist approach to BRCA risk that begins here could go a long way toward fostering a rhetoric of care. It could do this primarily by shifting how we think about BRCA+ women. As long as current feminist approaches to BRCA risk focus on the issue of compulsory choice, then we will be tempted to imagine BRCA+ women as disempowered people who need awareness or empowerment in order to make better (that is, freer) choices. But if there are no good choices, then perhaps we would be less likely to think in terms of this contrast between compulsory choice and free choice, and, further, if we are less likely to think in terms of this contrast, then perhaps we will also be less likely to think of BRCA+ women as disempowered. People who have no good choices are constrained, but they are not necessarily disempowered, and while they, too, need to be able to make better choices, it's not necessarily a lack of awareness or empowerment that's standing in their way.

Risk Is Real

I spent the entirety of the preceding chapter trying to demonstrate that BRCA risk is real by virtue of its enactment in cancer-screening practices, so why do I need to propose this idea as a rhetorical topic in this chapter? Indeed, the whole point of chapter 3 was to show that BRCA risk is real *so that* I could work toward a rhetoric of care for the at risk in this chapter. Why come back to this point now, at the end of chapter 4? I'll admit that this question has been a hard one for me to answer. At one point, early in my thinking about this book, I was mired in a bit of a chicken/egg dilemma: Do we need to understand risk as real so that we can have a rhetoric of care, or is the point of a rhetoric of care to give us ways of thinking, talking, and arguing about risk as something that is real? At first, I decided it was the former, that a rhetoric of care depends on our ability and willingness to acknowledge the realities of risk, and so that is how I proceeded, offering an explanation of that reality in chapter 3. But over the course of writing the book, I came to realize that this wasn't an either/or situation. Yes, a rhetoric of care depends on the idea that risk is real, but this idea should also be available to us as a resource for creating and promoting that rhetoric.

Risk Is Real in Rhetorics of Choice

To make this idea available to us in this way, though, we must first confront, as we did with some of the other topics presented here, the fact that it has been a key resource for creating and promoting the rhetoric of choice surrounding

BRCA risk. We might even say that it is the most fundamental assumption upon which that rhetoric rests. Within the rhetoric of choice, the reality of risk (understood, for instance, as the result of an altered, deleted, or added nucleotide in a gene on chromosome 17 or 13) is what demands that BRCA+ women make a choice, ideally one that will be based on knowledge and therefore capable of empowering them to take control of their health. Think back, for instance, to the advice from *Previvors* that I drew on in my discussion of product- and process-oriented views of BRCA risk. There, BRCA+ women are told that once they know they have a high risk of developing breast or ovarian cancer, they can either "do nothing" and "hope to beat the odds" or "take action" and try to "defy [. . . their] fate" (57). The notion of making a choice in order to defy one's fate smacks of the genetic determinism that has worried critics for decades and necessitated their counterarguments about the nonreality of risk, about how, as Ewald put it, nothing is a risk in itself but anything can become a risk depending on how one "analyzes the danger, considers the event" (199). Although arguments that take this social constructivist tact have sought to dismantle the rhetoric of choice surrounding BRCA risk, they have, as I argued in chapter 3, also provided us with another version of it. No matter which side of the issue we come down on, the free choice side or the compulsory choice side, we are still trafficking in the rhetoric of choice, still using that very common topic as our key rhetorical resource for making arguments about the quality of health care for BRCA+ women. In this sense, then, the idea that risk is real does a tremendous amount of work to secure and promote the circulation of rhetorics of choice, both explicitly in its demand that BRCA+ women make empowering choices to protect their health and implicitly in its solicitation of counterarguments that demonstrate the impossibility of making such choices freely.

Risk Is Real as "Ethos of Investigation"

So how, then, can we use this topic to promote a rhetoric of care? I want to begin answering this question by confronting another issue, namely that this topic comes closer than any other I've discussed to that gray area between the special topics and first principles, or *archai*. Aristotle drew attention to this gray area in the *Rhetoric*, noting that depending on what special topics a rhetor chose for a particular argument, he could end up moving out of rhetoric or dialectic and into the specialized knowledge of a particular subject matter "without its having been noticed" (1358a). While I recognize the potential for this kind of slippage (indeed, it is the source of the dilemma I describe above), I want to make the case here that we can use this topic in ways that keep us located within the realm of rhetoric. More specifically, I want to make the case that this topic offers us not just a proposition, that is, some material on which to build an argument, but also a disposition, a style of engagement, or, as Rose et al. say about governmentality, an "ethos of investigation" that by changing our relationship to rhetorics of choice can help foster a rhetoric of care (101). Of course, this is not a new idea, that the rhetorical function of the special topics is linked to ethos. Laura Wilder makes this point in *Rhetorical Strategies and Genre Conventions in Literary Studies*, writing that while the special topics help provide the means for building the logos of an argument, they also "subtly signal to other discourse community members that the writer has the credentials, or ethos, to make an argument worth regarding and tap into shared values, or pathos" (18). Fahnestock and Secor made the same point in their earlier study, "The Rhetoric of Literary Criticism," where they argued that the special topics are both the "constructs that enable scholars to operate" and the means by which they "manifest ethos" (91).

Arguably, though, to manifest a certain kind of ethos and to adopt a particular "ethos of investigation" are not exactly the same thing. The former is what we retrospectively observe when doing a topical analysis of discourse, while the latter is more like a strategy that we might adopt in order to engage in rhetorical invention. "Strategy," however, is not quite the right term, as it suggests a plan for achieving a preconceived result when what I wish to suggest, as indicated above, is something more akin to a disposition or style of engagement, a way of relating to or being in relation with the texts or discourses that matter to us. For an example of this notion of ethos, we might look back to Muckelbauer and his effort to shift from the extraction of constants to the extraction of singular rhythms through the "inclination" or "pragmatic character" of scholarly engagement. Muckelbauer tried to implement this shift in his own engagement with rhetorical theory by following five "stylistic rules" or principles: the principle of generosity, of not orienting toward intentions, of selective reading, of connectivity, and of nonrecognition. While none of these principles provided Muckelbauer with a plan for extracting singular rhythms, they did position or dispose him in such a way that it would be harder to extract constants. Take, for instance, the last of his of "stylistic rules," the principle of nonrecognition. Although Muckelbauer's work is deeply indebted to theorists like Nietzsche, Derrida, and Deleuze, he does not often quote from or summarize their texts (*Future of Invention* 47). On the one hand, this nonrecognition stems from Muckelbauer's belief that their influence is so great that to cite them often would seem "disingenuous," implying that their work is somehow "outside" of him (47). But on the other hand, the point of such nonrecognition is to reconfigure one's relationship to a text in such a way as to not be responsible for explaining what it means, thus opening up, in his estimation, more opportunities for seeing what it can *do*.

This kind of reconfiguration, I submit, is what we stand to gain by employing the idea that risk is real as a rhetorical topic. Importantly, the point of such a move would not be to make arguments about the reality of risk (that is, to use this topic as a first principle) or to be more persuasive rhetors by demonstrating our solidarity with BRCA+ women (that is, to make a more traditional appeal to ethos)—though I think both of these efforts would fit in just fine with the goals of a rhetoric of care. The point, rather, would be to comport ourselves to the discourses surrounding BRCA risk in such a way that we are not automatically tasked with the work of distinguishing reality from appearance. This is what happens within a constructivist orientation where our relationship to those discourses is engineered by suspicion.[13] Positioned as the debunker, we are obligated to determine how something that isn't real has been made to seem real, and who, on account of this sleight of hand, has been disadvantaged or disempowered. As Latour argues in the 2010 essay, "An Attempt at a 'Compositionist Manifesto,'" such positioning has yielded a great deal of "productive energy," but it has also had the "immense drawback of creating a massive gap between what [. . . is] felt and what [. . . is] real" (475). He addresses what is at stake in creating such a gap in his earlier *Reassembling the Social*, arguing that we should not be surprised that enthusiasm for demonstrating the social construction of scientific facts has been met "with such fury by the actors themselves" (92). To wit:

> For physicists, it is far from the same thing to settle complex controversies about black holes or to be presented instead with 'power struggles among physicists.' For a religious soul, it is far from the same thing to address God in prayer and to be said to pray only to the "personalization of Society." For a lawyer, it is not the same thing to obey the Constitution or to yield to powerful lobbies hidden behind the law. For a haute couture seamstress, it is not the same thing to cut through thick and shiny velvet or to be said to make a "social distinction visible." For a follower of a cult, it's not the same thing to be tied to the existence of a divinity and to be told that one adores a fetish made out of wood. (92–93)

Might we add to this list that for BRCA+ women it is far from the same thing to have a bilateral salpingo-oophorectomy in order to avoid ovarian cancer as it is to legitimate gynecology as a medical specialization? Or that to undergo an intense cancer-screening regimen on account of a positive BRCA mutation test is not the same thing as to submit to neoliberal forms of self-government or ideologies of genetic determinism? Or, pushing the point even further, that to have a bilateral mastectomy in order to be alive to have and raise children is not the same thing as to conform to heterosexist gender norms about female bodies and maternal responsibilities? And if we can make these additions, granting BRCA risk a place among other irreducible objects like black holes, thick and shiny velvet, and the Constitution, then can we also find different ways of comporting ourselves in relation to the BRCA-related issues and discourses that matter to us and those at risk? Using this topic in this way won't necessarily diminish its function within the discourses of BRCA+ women, meaning that belief in the indisputable, unified, and nonsocial reality of risk will continue to elicit rhetorics of choice in those discourses, but it can reduce the circulation of those rhetorics within our own work, opening up more space for a rhetoric of care.

Space for a Rhetoric of Care

Opening up space for a rhetoric of care is a laudable goal. In fact, in name it might seem so laudable that we can't argue against it. Who can be against *care*? But the fact is that plenty of people who care about BRCA+ women and the issues they face will find these topics and the premises on which they are based troubling. They will worry, for instance, that what I've done here is provide another "cover" for genetic determinism or hereditarian ideologies. Or that a rhetoric of care is just one more inducement for women to submit to biomedicine and the ways in which it tries to control their bodies. Relatedly, they might worry that I have further muddied the line between health and illness, making it even more likely that those with genetic mutations will be thought of (and will think of themselves) as the "presymptomatically ill" or the "worried well." To a degree, I think these are legitimate concerns, which is to say that I think they offer us valuable insights into the problems of genetic medicine and any attempt, like mine, to normalize its presence in our lives. But if these insights are valuable, then they are also incomplete and not as revelatory as they once seemed to be, meaning that they are not doing the critical or ameliorative work we thought they would. BRCA risk is as hybrid an object as we can imagine. It cannot be purified to either nature or culture, and so it illustrates, as much as any of the examples offered by Latour, why we have to redirect our critical efforts, working more on the task of assembling than debunking, on giving the participants an arena in which to gather rather than on lifting the rug from beneath their feet ("Why Has Critique Run Out of Steam?" 226).

As I said earlier, the topics I've presented here are no panacea for solving the problems created by rhetorics of choice. However, I do think they offer us a way to begin engaging in this redirection of our critical efforts, in building some "arenas," as Latour puts it, for those who find themselves having to participate in and interact with the messy object of BRCA risk. Of course, to suggest, as I just did, that these topics are ways of building arenas, not the arenas themselves (to stick with Latour's metaphor) is to highlight another important difference between my efforts here and Mol's in *The Logic of Care*. Whereas she offers readers an alternative logic, one that tries to define good care in the context of diabetes on its own terms, I have not offered an alternative rhetoric in this chapter but rather have tried to craft from the biosocial discourses surrounding BRCA risk a set of topoi that might be used as a tool for building such a rhetoric. Yes, I believe that we are both participating in the inventive mode of inquiry that I described in the first part of this chapter, but I haven't used that mode of inquiry as she did to describe care in detail or to say what makes it good in the context of BRCA risk. This is the work that remains to be done, the work of figuring out what arguments we can make about care in this context if we use different conceptual starting places, assuming, for instance, that clinical risk assessments are real but not unified or indisputable, that a lack of good choices is constraining but not necessarily disempowering, or that health is more than the absence of disease, even in the case of genetic risk. These are just possibilities, and to be sure, there are others. What I hope to have demonstrated here is that we can read the rhetorics of choice surrounding BRCA risk productively, using them to create tools, some heuristics, that might help move our minds out of their "habitual grooves" and shake them free from "a stereotypic past that wants to be retrieved."

Conclusion | Invention in RSTM: Another Moderate Response to the Two-World Problem

When Richard Young described heuristics in those terms, as something capable of moving the mind out of its "habitual grooves, of shaking it loose from a stereotypic past that wants to be retrieved," he likely would not have imagined them showing up almost four decades later in the context of RSTM scholarship. Indeed, RSTM was not a well-established area of inquiry when Young wrote "Arts, Crafts, Gifts, and Knacks," the 1980 essay in which this description of heuristics appeared. In that essay, Young was concerned with the teaching of writing or, more specifically, with the teaching of one aspect of writing, invention. His goal was to use the new classicist understanding of the term *techne* (or art, as he referred to it) to explain and legitimize the teaching of invention in the composition classroom. That a scholar like Young would turn to the ancient concept of *techne* as a way to achieve this goal is unsurprising. *Techne* offered him and other likeminded scholars a viable alternative to competing romanticist notions of art. If, in their view, those romanticist notions left invention unknowable and unteachable, a mysterious gift that could be encouraged but not directly cultivated,[1] then the new classicist understanding offered a different path, one where the processes of discovery were generalizable enough for researchers to study and for instructors to teach. Moreover, for more than 2,500 years, the term *techne* had been synonymous with making, that is, with bringing into existence those things that could either be or not be, and so the resonance between it and invention, between a kind of knowledge meant to yield useful (but not permanently so) results and the rhetorical processes of discovery, must have been compelling.

Almost forty years later, I believe that this resonance remains compelling, although for significantly different reasons. As I have argued throughout this book, giving objects their due means redirecting our critical capacities, engaging them in such a way as to care for and protect, not debunk. This, of course, is how Latour frames the challenge we face, mildly admonishing us in "Why Has

Critique Run Out of Steam?" to be at least as critical and reflective about our intellectual equipment as good generals have to be about their military equipment (231). We must "retest the linkages," he warns, and be willing to "revise from scratch the whole paraphernalia" if they don't hold up. While I think it's safe to say that many of those linkages have failed us, I don't believe that we, as rhetoricians, are in a position of having to revise from scratch our "whole paraphernalia." In fact, I believe that insofar as our "paraphernalia" includes an understanding of rhetorical invention as productive art or *techne*, we have precisely the kinds of intellectual equipment that these new challenges demand. I tried to demonstrate this in chapter 4 by offering a set of topics designed to help foster a rhetoric of care for those at genetic risk of breast and ovarian cancers due to a BRCA mutation. Here, in these concluding pages, I want to address the implications of that demonstration (and the argument I based it on) by placing it in conversation with related efforts in RSTM scholarship and acknowledging some of its limitations.

To begin, though, a brief review. In chapter 4, I offered readers four rhetorical topics that I framed as ways of changing rather than explaining the biosocial and critical discourses surrounding BRCA risk. I aligned this distinction between changing and explaining with rhetoric's inventive and interpretive (or heuristic and hermeneutic) functions respectively and acknowledged not only the difficulty of maintaining it, that is, of operating in a purely inventive mode, but also the fact that invention had helped to create exactly the problem I was responding to, that of an overreliance on constructivist critique. The challenge, then, was to articulate a version of invention that was non-epistemological in orientation, one that would not so easily facilitate such critique and thus could work with the new materialist theory, even if it wasn't built from it. To do this, I turned first to the work of Richard McKeon, aligning my effort to create new topics from the biosocial discourses surrounding BRCA risk with his understanding of rhetoric as an architectonic productive art. While I recognized the impossibility of emptying such an understanding of rhetoric of its epistemological implications, I tried to mitigate them by drawing on Aristotle's description of productive knowledge in *Nicomachean Ethics*, as well as Janet Atwill's commentary on that description in *Rhetoric Reclaimed*, in order to highlight the instrumental nature of *technics*, that is, the fact that it is a kind of making or bringing forth whose products are meant to help their users *do* something rather than *know* something. I compared this distinction between doing and knowing to the one John Law makes between construction and enactment, arguing that because the latter of these two metaphors better described the art of rhetoric, constructivist critique was something of a mismatch, an intellectual exercise better suited for inscriptions meant to describe or tell than for enactments meant to intervene or to "make a difference in a body or a life," as Law put it. I further elaborated this argument through the work of John Muckelbauer, whose efforts to rethink rhetorical invention in relation to the problem of negation pushed the distinction between doing and knowing one step further, even as it also explained why that distinction could never be complete. For Muckelbauer, the goal of invention was not just to see how a text performs (or, even less, to explain what it means) but rather to make it perform by reading it productively. Put differently, the goal wasn't just recognizing texts as enactments but actually enacting them, using them to ask new questions, to make new connections, and to think differently about the problems that perplexed us. Finally, I suggested that by trying to make texts perform, to enact them in such a way that invention itself became the objective, we had come back to McKeon's understanding of rhetoric as an architectonic productive art, provided that we took into account my efforts to mitigate its epistemological implications.

So where do all of these comparisons and connections leave us? What good are they outside of the specific context of my argument about BRCA risk? To answer these questions, I want to turn to S. Scott Graham's 2015 *The Politics of Pain Medicine: A Rhetorical-Ontological Inquiry*, a book that I referenced in the introduction and then again briefly in chapter 3. Broadly speaking, Graham's book is an effort to respond to the "two-world" problem, that is, the nature/culture or subject/object divide, that has haunted not just critical theory in the humanities and social sciences but also the subject of his study: pain medicine and science. Graham does this through a form of "rhetorical-ontological" inquiry wherein he analyzes the representational practices that members of the Midwest Pain Group use to calibrate various diagnostic ontologies and bring them together in such a way as to foster the emergence of nonmodern or hybrid models of pain that reject the centuries-old understanding of pain as either a mental *or* a physical phenomena (65). Through his analysis of the MPG's "off-label" discussions, for instance, Graham identifies four functional stases and tracks their relationships to each other and the various topical resolutions that emerged from them, showing how members used these rhetorical devices to foster the kind of "discursive transformations" necessary for establishing nonmodern pain ontologies (116). Other parts of his project focus on different rhetorical features, warranting topoi and trope shifting, for instance, but in each

case Graham's goal is to offer a rhetorical-ontological investigation of the discursive space of the MPG that can explain how "representational activity circu-
lates within and contributes to the deeper ecology of practices in which those
acts of representation are embedded" (69). Alongside (and, indeed, through)
this explanation, Graham also makes the case rhetoric and STS need to work
together, showing how each field has reached a point of "theoretical symmetry"
through its embrace of the new materialisms (12).

   In addition to this argument about the relationship between rhetoric and
STS, one of the strengths of *The Politics of Pain Medicine* is how carefully Graham reflects on the implications of this response to the two-world problem,
particularly the ways in which it butts up against the more antirepresentationalist strains of new materialist theory and what this conflict means for rhetoricians who recognize the need to acknowledge the agency of the material, but
who don't want to reject all inquiry into representation (204). Graham elaborates this dilemma in his concluding chapter, "Finding the Groove," arguing that
the postmodern critique of modernism and the new materialist response to that
critique are both hypercorrections, that is, hard turns meant to undo what had
come before (204). In the case of the postmodern critique of modernism, evidence of that overcorrection lies in the epistemic and hegemonic fallacies that I
described in the introduction, while in the case of the new materialist response,
it lies in what Graham describes as a "hostility toward inquiry into representation" that can make new materialist theory "very foreign to rhetoricians" (83).
What Graham means by "hostility" here isn't so much the kind of "innocuous"
questioning of the linguistic turn, hermeneutics, or genealogical critique that we
see in the work of scholars like Coole and Frost, Bennett, or Latour but rather
a harder line antirepresentationalism that rejects any inquiry into the symbolic
as inappropriate and undesirable (83). Offering the "transmission model" of
communication posited by Levi Bryant in *The Democracy of Objects* as an example
of such antirepresentationalism, Graham argues that any rhetorical theory or
inquiry grounded in this strain of new materialism cannot "move one iota beyond
the ludic postmodernism" that it purportedly rejects (83). In other words, it
cannot productively respond to the two-world problem because by always privileging the object over the subject, it works to reinscribe it (18). Thus, the goal for
Graham (and, in his view, for rhetoric studies in general) is to provide a more
"moderate" response to the two-world problem, a response that is less a hard
turn and more of a "tweaking of the wheel" that can move us "back to the center" where we can "balance out the opposing pressure systems that demand either

object-oriented or human centered accounts" (204). This is how he positions his own form of rhetorical-ontological inquiry, praxiography of representation, writing that while he accepts "the new materialist move away from representation," he's not willing to "throw the baby out with the bathwater" and abandon all inquiry into representation. After all, new materialist analysis is about doing rather than seeing or knowing, and what is language (in the view of rhetoricians) if not a way of doing (83–84)?

One way, then, to understand the implications of the arguments I've made in *Being at Genetic Risk* is to see them as another moderate response to the two-world problem, that is, as an attempt, like Graham's, to take seriously the challenges posed by new materialist theory without abandoning all inquiry into the symbolic. In this sense, we might say that *Being at Genetic Risk* offers another version of the kind of rhetorical-ontological inquiry that demonstrates the need for rhetoric and STS to work together. Indeed, even though I do not argue that rhetoric and STS need each other in the way that Graham does, evidence of that need is apparent in the book's structure and arguments, particularly in chapter 3's praxiographic inquiry into BRCA risk and the fact that I frame this inquiry as a prerequisite for moving toward a rhetoric of care. If we could not understand BRCA risk as something that is real despite and, in fact, because of its messy, "highly uncertain and loudly disputed" nature, then we would remain locked, I worried, in a kind of constructivist critique that promoted a rhetoric of choice even as it argued that free choice was an illusion. Making this case for the reality of BRCA risk, though, was not primarily a task for rhetorical inquiry, at least not as we have typically understood it. I needed to read my data referentially, as Mak did in her study of hermaphroditism, in order to follow BRCA risk through the high-risk breast cancer–screening practices that enact it. And while I believe that this kind of reading offers lessons for rhetoricians, for instance, that praxiography can be conducted through alternative "empirical access points," including texts, I also believe that it is primarily the province of STS, at least as I have executed and presented it here. Unlike Graham, I did not adapt praxiography into a rhetorical methodology. Rather, I tried to show how praxiography could be conducted by rhetoricians, and I did this *because I needed to*, that is, because my efforts to intervene into the problem of choice in the biosocial and critical discourses surrounding BRCA risk depended on it. However, to the degree that those efforts, which are primarily the province of rhetoric, constitute the heart of my argument in *Being at Genetic Risk*, they demonstrate that this dependence is mutual, that my praxiographic inquiry into

BRCA risk alone could not have provided an adequate response to the problem of choice.

Even if we agree that my work here offers another version of rhetorical-ontological inquiry (and thus another example of how rhetoric and STS need each other), though, we must acknowledge that it isn't the same kind of "inquiry into representation" that Graham offers in *The Politics of Pain Medicine*. In fact, more than the kind of inquiry that Graham *offers*, I would argue that it is an example of the kind he *calls for*, namely a "more fully interventional" form of rhetorical-ontological inquiry (215). In the concluding pages of *The Politics of Pain Medicine*, Graham identifies two future directions for rhetorical-ontological inquiry. The first is an increased focus on the "reciprocal relationship between words and things," or, more to the point, a willingness to understand words as things (208, 212). In arguing that we should understand words as things, Graham joins those who advocate for a kind of flat ontology (or "symmetry" in the parlance of ANT) where things, defined in Heidegger's terms as gatherings, are not ontologically distinct, even if they gather through very different mechanisms, for instance, through "blood flow and radioactive decay" on the one hand, and "algorithms and images" on the other (212). The advantage of this line of inquiry, in Graham's view, is that it avoids the rhetoric-as-epiphenomenon problem characteristic of the more antirepresentationalist strains of new materialism ("Object-Oriented Ontology's Binary Duplication" 121). His second recommendation, which is the one I focus on here, stems from a concern that even as a praxiography of representation shifts our attention from what language means to what it does, the product it yields is an account, that is, a representation, whose own ontology falls into the category that Graham dubs "empirical-discursive" (*Politics of Pain Medicine* 212). As he puts it, praxiography of representation "involves an iterative series of ocular and inscriptive practices so as to create an account of doings" (212), and while Mol argues in *The Body Multiple* that such accounts are themselves interventions, Graham remains concerned about their limitations as representations, acknowledging their potential to commit epistemic violence and thus calling for forms of rhetorical-ontological inquiry that can use their "investigational resources to catalyze and assist interventional and emancipatory projects in a wide variety of domains" (215).

The topics that I offered in chapter 4 are representations that fall into the same ontological category as the products of Graham's praxiography of representation, the empirical-discursive category. Thus, we could never say they are incapable of the kind of epistemic violence Graham worries about. However, insofar as they are not primarily an "account" of language's "doings" but rather an attempt to make language *do something*, they offer one example of what a "more fully interventional" form of rhetorical-ontological inquiry might look like. As Mol did in *The Logic of Care*, I tried to work with my materials "the way an artist works with paint or with tissue and thread" (10), that is, by using them to make something, in this case, a set of topics that could be used to change rather than just explain the critical and biosocial discourses surrounding BRCA risk. Of course, we use language all the time to change things, even when we are "just" explaining (and, for the record, I have done plenty of explaining in this book). For this reason, I find the phrasing of Graham's call very felicitous. He asks for a "more fully" interventional form of inquiry, suggesting that the difference he's after is one of degree, not kind. In my view, this is precisely what an approach to invention built through the work of McKeon, Atwill, and Muckelbauer gives us, an architectonic form of inquiry where the goal is invention itself, where rheto-ric is not just a means of creating (or analyzing) argument through various "schemata and devices," as McKeon put it, but a means of creating those "sche-mata and devices." Like McKeon, I have focused on rhetorical topics here, but our efforts do not have to be limited to this particular rhetorical device. In addi-tion, we might work on the introduction of new tropes, as Leah Ceccarelli did in her 2013 book, *On the Frontier of Science: An American Rhetoric of Exploration and Exploitation*. Here, Ceccarelli examines the history and rhetorical entail-ments of the frontier metaphor that has long guided the public discourse of American scientists, demonstrating that part of its function has been to narrow "our perception of who is qualified to undertake scientific research (ruggedly individualistic men), the motives that guide scientists (progressive), the means and proper actions they take to achieve their goals (competitive and exploit-ative), and the setting in which they work (unclaimed territory)" (3–4). How-ever, rather than simply denouncing this function of the metaphor in the hopes that scientists will stop using it, Ceccarelli identifies other metaphors that might modify or mitigate its effects, for instance the "biopirate" metaphor that has been used to highlight "the complexity of ownership claims over the biological 'wealth' discovered by scientific researchers," the landmine metaphor that has been used to suggest that scientific fronts are filled with dangers as well as promises, and the scientist-as-detective metaphor that could be used to high-light the importance of puzzle-solving skills in science (150). While Ceccarelli is clear about the fact that these alternative metaphors are not perfect, she does see in them opportunities for crafting more sophisticated public understandings of American science.

Marita Gronnvoll and Jamie Landau demonstrated a similar approach to metaphor criticism three years earlier in "From Viruses to Russian Roulette to Dance: A Rhetorical Critique and Creation of Genetic Metaphors," the 2010 essay in which they argued for an "orientation to rhetorical criticism" built on Robert Ivie's call to identify the "untapped potential" of dysfunctional metaphors and to create more productive replacements (47–48). Particularly in their pursuit of this second objective, to create more productive replacement metaphors, Gronnvoll and Landau demonstrate an architectonic approach to rhetorical invention, identifying promising but latent or underdeveloped elements of lay discourses about genetics and working them into two metaphors (that of a dance and of a band) better suited for highlighting the "physically collaborative" relationship between genes and the environment (65). Hoping that these new metaphors might motivate people to "create environments that are health protecting, avoid environments that are health destroying, and work in other ways on a daily basis to improve their health," Gronvoll and Landau advocate for their inclusion in public service announcements, health campaign materials, and other media messages (48).

Although Gronvoll and Landau do believe in and advocate for the ability of their replacement metaphors to effect positive change, they, like Cecarelli, acknowledge the challenges that any inclusion or application of the tropes would face. First, there is no guarantee that they would actually be used. New metaphors, even those designed with ameliorative aims, are not always persuasive and so they might not be readily incorporated into lay or public health discourses (64). Moreover, even if they are incorporated, they are not conceptually perfect alternatives, and so they could cause new problems or further entrench existing ones (66). The same limitations apply here, to the topics I've offered as a response to the problem of choice, and, presumably, to any effort to engage in this type of architectonic, rhetorical-ontological inquiry. Creating new "schemata and devices" is one thing. Their having any discernible effects in people's lives is another. And even if they do have an effect, even if, for instance, a topic like being between the devil and the deep can help foster a rhetoric of care where to be constrained is not necessarily to be disempowered, we must recognize that this achievement would not be as "fully interventional" as, say, a more accurate way of assessing cancer risk or a method of breast MRI that had perfect sensitivity and specificity. But neither this recognition nor any of the limitations mentioned here should deter us from the work of rhetorical invention in RSTM. Yes, we may need STS (or other allied fields), and yes, new materialist theory may be curtailing rhetoric's epistemological capacities, but it has also provided the impetus for envisioning new capacities, as in the case of Graham's argument that we should understand words as things, and for rethinking old ones, as in the case of my argument that *techne*, the paradigm of productive knowledge, provides a way of understanding rhetorical invention architectonically, but in the terms of enactment rather than construction.

This argument, of course, is no panacea for solving the two-world problem, just as the topics presented in chapter 4 were no panacea for solving the problem of choice in the discourses surrounding BRCA risk. But both, I think, offer a way forward when there is not only a recognized need within RSTM for rhetoric to contribute more than just analysis to the problems that beset and perplex us (Scott et al. 2) but also a broader call from quarters outside of rhetoric for a reconsideration of what critical engagement in the social sciences and humanities should look like and what it should try to accomplish. I've relied heavily in this book on Latour's work to explain that call, turning frequently (perhaps too frequently) to his claim that we have to stop trying to pull the rug from beneath the feet of the naïve believers and instead give the participants new arenas in which to gather. But if I have relied too heavily on this characteristically colorful claim of Latour's, then that is because I believe it resonates so strongly with what rhetoric can do when "just" analysis isn't sufficient. Yes, analysis is important—essential, even. And rhetoric has demonstrated well its efficacy in that mode of critical engagement. But it can also provide us with some of the tools necessary for building those arenas and for giving the participants, who are not naïve in their beliefs, new places to gather.

Notes

Introduction

1. As I explain in chapter 1, BRCA mutations are not the only ones responsible for inherited susceptibility to breast and ovarian cancers. Moreover, women can have inherited susceptibility to these cancers without having any known genetic mutation. Thus, the broader term used to describe this susceptibility is Hereditary Breast and Ovarian Cancer (HBOC) syndrome. I decided to focus my study on women with identified BRCA mutations because the clinical guidelines for them, that is, for managing BRCA risk related to a BRCA1 or BRCA2 mutation, are clearer and better established. However, the arguments that I make in this book can apply more broadly to anyone with HBOC syndrome.

2. I use this term, "BRCA risk," throughout the book to refer to inherited susceptibility to breast and ovarian cancers due to an identified BRCA1 or BRCA2 mutation.

3. For an excellent examination of the limits of the hermeneutics of suspicion within literary studies, see Rita Felski's 2015 *Limits of Critique*, especially chapter 2, "The Stakes of Suspicion," which considers the history of suspicion as a mood and a mode of scholarly engagement. Among other things, Felski shows how suspicion sets up a binary system in which not being suspicious automatically means being subservient or oppressed (51). Within this system, she argues, "[w]hatever is not critique, by contrast, must fall into the camp of the credulous, compliant, and co-opted. In short, critique requires its antithesis in order to shore up its own virtues: the foil of a crushing system of domination or subjugation that turns out, nonetheless, to be strangely vulnerable to the threat of verbal exposure" (50).

4. FORCE does serve men and women, as both can inherit and be affected by BRCA mutations. In this study, however, I focus only on women with BRCA mutations because they make up the overwhelming majority of the biosocial community surrounding BRCA risk, meaning that most of the discourse in that community is written by or about women, addressing the specific medical issues they face as BRCA carriers, for instance, not just risk for breast cancer but also ovarian cancer.

5. See Alcorn's *Changing the Subject in English Class* and Rickert's *Acts of Enjoyment*.

6. See, for instance, Thomas Rickert's *Ambient Rhetoric*; S. Scott Graham's *Politics of Pain Medicine*; Scot Barnett and Casey Boyle's *Rhetoric Through Everyday Things*; and Scot Barnett's *Rhetorical Realism*.

Chapter 1

1. For sources that identify choice as a key (but also illusory) marker of difference between eugenics and the new genetics, see Kerr et al.'s "Eugenics and the New Genetics in Britain" and Alan Petersen's "Scope and Context of the New Genetics." Petersen, for instance, claims that for "proponents of the new genetics, the word 'new' acts as a boundary marker, delineating that which promotes individual 'freedom of choice' (and is therefore assumed to be necessarily 'good') from that which denotes coercive control (and is therefore deemed 'bad')" (40).

He further argues that unlike eugenics, "which is focused on some members of the population with the aim of eliminating 'undesirables' (negative eugenics) or breeding of the fit (positive eugenics), the new genetics is seen to present positive options and to allow individuals to make their own 'informed' voluntary decisions. This is facilitated through 'nondirective' genetic counseling, which is frequently presented as the hallmark of the new genetics" (41).

2. See Chen and Parmigiana's "Meta-Analysis of BRCA1 and BRCA2 Penetrance," where they report that approximately 20 to 30 percent of BRCA carriers never get breast cancer, and 35 to 85 percent do not get ovarian cancer.

3. There are two main ways of referring to these surgeries: (1) prophylactic bilateral mastectomy and prophylactic bilateral salpingo-oophorectomy; and (2) risk-reducing bilateral mastectomy and risk-reducing bilateral salpingo-oophorectomy. In general, the modifier "risk-reducing" is preferred because it is a better acknowledgment of the fact that these surgeries are not completely protective, meaning they do not completely eliminate cancer risk. However, many people still use the term "prophylactic," especially in the common abbreviations "PBM" and "PBSO." My use of these terms changes with the sources I am working with.

4. In an essay for *Nature Education*, Sarah Sabatinos explains that DNA replication is a complicated process that begins at predetermined DNA sequences known as "replication origins." Once the process begins, DNA replication proteins organize into a structure called the "replication fork," which is where DNA "unwinding" and synthesizing happen. The replication fork, in other words, is where the double helix structure of DNA begins to open up, creating two strands (which can look like two prongs of a fork) that will be used as the basis for generating duplicate copies of the DNA molecule. But a variety of "impediments" can stall this process of duplication, making the replication fork one of the key sites for DNA damage that can lead to mutation or cell death.

5. While BRCA mutations are associated most directly with breast and ovarian cancers, they can also affect one's risk of other cancers—endometrial, pancreatic, prostate in the case of BRCA1, and prostate, pancreatic, and melanoma in the case of BRCA2 (Bougie and Weberpals 2).

6. See Couch et al.'s "Two Decades After BRCA," a 2014 study of "sequence variants" in BRCA mutations.

7. The NCCN guidelines do not include a recommendation for ovarian cancer screening because neither transvaginal ultrasound nor serum CA-125 testing have been shown to be sufficiently sensitive or specific enough to be effective. However, the guidelines note that these tests may be considered at the clinician's discretion starting at age thirty to thirty-five years ("NCCN Guidelines").

8. The closest thing to an exception in this situation is the NCCN recommendation that BRCA+ women have PBSO by ages thirty to thirty-five (BRCA1) or forty to forty-five (BRCA2).

9. For an explanation and critique of nondirectiveness, see Alan Petersen's "Facilitating Autonomy," particularly pages 135–58.

10. The discourse from the FORCE message boards comes from the posts that I sampled for chapter 3's praxiographic inquiry into BRCA risk. For details about how I sampled those posts, see endnote 5 of chapter 3. The interviews I reference here were conducted in late 2014 and early 2015 and were also part of my research for chapter 3. I briefly draw on them here because they illustrate well several features of the rhetoric of choice, especially characterizations of knowledge as the key to empowerment.

11. While I do believe that this is true, that broad ethical and biopolitical changes affect lay discourses about genetics, I fully agree with Celeste Condit's argument in *The Meanings of the Gene* that it's better to think of those discourses in terms of rhetorical formations (rather

than Foucault's discursive formations) that are always contested and formed by "multiple related but independent components" (253). The utility of thinking in these terms in the case of BRCA risk is borne out by, among other things, the fact that rhetorics of genetic determinism coexist with rhetorics of choice. See also my "Genetic Subjectivity *in situ*."

Chapter 2

1. Constructivist approaches to risk have been productive in other areas besides genetic risk. Take, for instance, J. Blake Scott's 2003 *Risky Rhetoric*. Here Scott critically analyzes the discourses surrounding HIV antibody testing, showing how rhetorical features in these discourses have a disciplinary function that aims more at shaping subjectivities to be in line with dominant cultural norms than at improving outcomes for those at risk of HIV. Another more recent example of the productiveness of this approach is Marika Seigel's 2013 *Rhetoric of Pregnancy*, a book that demonstrates how pregnancy manuals and how-to guides discipline women's bodies. Seigel does this in a chapter on risk, for instance, by arguing that the risk assessment approach taken by pregnancy manuals discourages pregnant women from challenging the status quo and teaches them to manage their risky bodies in order to produce a normal baby.

2. See, for instance, Condit's *The Meanings of the Gene*; Rose's *The Politics of Life Itself*; and Hedgecoe's "Reconstructing Geneticization" and "Ethical Boundary Work."

3. A good example of this type of critique, i.e., one that tries to move away from the language-as-epiphenomenon theory implicit in Marxist versions of ideology (as well as the radical constructivism that gets posited as its alternative) but whose actual analysis still pivots around an appearance/reality distinction, is Hasain's *Rhetoric of Eugenics in Anglo-American Thought*. See especially chapter 7, "The Return of Eugenics: Ideographic Fragments and the Mythology of the Human Genome Project."

4. Rose's *Politics of Life Itself* is a compelling example of such an analysis. This doesn't mean that Rose's text is problem free. His argument tends to paint the new genetics in the very broad brushstrokes of opportunity versus destiny or optimism versus fatalism, overlooking the ways in which rhetorics of genetic determinism still operate in the discourses of the genetically at risk. But despite this, Rose makes a strong case for leaving social critique behind in order to better account for the ways in which those at risk construct themselves as active, enterprising subjects in order to manage genetic risk and live good lives. In this sense, his work illustrates well the attempt within governmentality studies to take programs at face value rather than peeling back their surface to identify hidden political forces.

5. This point highlights a distinction between my argument and the one that Latour makes in "Why Has Critique Run Out of Steam?" Latour argues that we need to retool and move past (or radically rethink) constructivist forms of critique not only because they have become predictable, repetitive, and ineffective (which is my argument, too) but also because they've fallen into the "wrong hands," which is to say that they've been turned against us in order to create what he terms "artificially maintained scientific controversy" (226). This means, for instance, that now arguments about the social construction of science and lack of scientific certainty are being used to challenge the "real objective and incontrovertible facts" about things like climate change, putting us, critics in the humanities and social sciences, in the position of having to defend "good matters of fact" from the illusion that they are nothing but "bad ideological biases" (227). While I do think constructivist critiques of genetic risk have gone on for so long that it's (too) easy to consider naïve anyone who believes that mutations are real, I do not believe that those critiques amount to or result in an artificially maintained scientific controversy.

6. This is, of course, the Marxist definition of ideology as false consciousness, which is often understood in terms of the idea, which Marx expressed in *Capital*, that "they do not know it, but they are doing it." Theories of ideology have evolved beyond this version—due, in large part, to an effort to revise the oversimplified theory of subjectivity on which it is based (namely the idea that the knowledge produced via critique will change belief and belief, in turn, will change action). But as I point out, in terms of its use as a hermeneutic tool, this version of ideology has been and still is very commonly deployed in critiques of genetic risk.

7. Lippman is more explicit about the ideological nature of the process of geneticization in her 1998, "Politics of Health."

8. Happe makes this constructivist position most clear in her concluding chapter, "Toward a Biosociality Without Genes," where she writes that genetic risk "is not something the scientist or physician discovers but is a rhetorical construction, one that articulates a particular configuration of relations between patients, institutions, and industrial capitalism" (178). Further, in summarizing her overall point that "scientific objects and medical practices are inextricably tied to the world outside the laboratory and the physician's office," she argues that "[n]ature does not produce the normal and the pathological; social discourses (including that of science) do. [...] Genes and the bodies they inhabit, moreover, come to the researcher and the doctor already inscribed by the social. They are symbolic as much as they are material; indeed, how bodies 'matter' is very much a product of discourse. No object of scientific investigation or medical intervention comes to us ready made but is, rather, the produce of interest-driven discourse" (178–79).

9. See, for instance, Bradbury et al.'s "Uptake and Timing of Bilateral Salpingo-Oophorectomy Among BRCA1 and BRCA2 Mutation Carriers."

10. Happe does not explain how the risk associated with BRCA mutations is socially constructed (an omission that illustrates how ingrained and self-evident this argument has become) but rather notes, in an endnote, that it has been demonstrated by Beck's 1992 *Risk Society*, a text known more for its wavering between a weak realist and a weak constructivist approach to risk than for really demonstrating its socially constructed nature (Lupton, *Risk and Sociocultural Theory* 59–60). Indeed, some risk scholars opt for the governmentality approach to risk over the risk society approach precisely because the former takes a stronger constructivist perspective.

11. See also Lupton's "Risk as Moral Danger"; Petersen and Bunton's *Foucault*, particularly the essays by Nettleton and Bunton; Petersen and Bunton's *New Genetics and the Public's Health*; and Bunton and Petersen's *Genetic Governance*.

12. In his 2003, "Governmentality, Critical Scholarship, and the Medical Humanities," Petersen explicitly calls for the kind of merger between social critique and governmentality studies that characterizes his own scholarship. Specifically, he argues that in order for governmentality studies to become more politically radical, they will have to "forge a more fruitful dialogue" with forms of sociological inquiry that have been more interesting in generalizing and theory building (199).

13. For another governmentality-based study that identifies the ways in which certain discourses "responsibilize" women at risk of breast cancer, see Robertson's "Embodying Risk, Embodying Political Rationality."

14. Both Crabb and LeCouteur and Dubriwny are clear about their constructivist view of risk. In an endnote, Crabb and LeCouteur draw on Lupton and Petersen (and, by proxy, Castel and Ewald) to argue that the dangers we have come to understand as risks are better understood as socially and historically constructed than as objective entities that can inform rational decision making (17). Dubriwny turns to Mitchell Dean (which is also by proxy a turn to Ewald) to explain that she understands risk from the perspective of governmentality as a means of ordering reality rather than reality itself (27–28).

Chapter 3

1. A good example of a study in rhetoric and technical communication that acknowledges the reality of risk (at least implicitly) but does not embrace a kind of naïve realism is Beverly Sauer's 2003 *The Rhetoric of Risk*. Sauer's book does not directly address the nature of risk per se, but instead it takes a rhetorical approach to risk by studying the problem of documentation in the hazardous environments of mining. Sauer shows where in the cycle of technical documentation uncertainties arise and how those uncertainties can be better dealt with by including embodied forms of knowledge like speech and gesture.

2. The distinction Law is referring to here between ontological and epistemological terms applies to approaches to studies of public understanding of science (for instance, what publics *do* versus what they *know*), not to the differences between ANT- and enactment-inspired versions of STS, both of which would be considered "ontological."

3. BRCA+ women can participate in other practices to reduce their risk of developing cancer, for instance, limiting alcohol intake and exercising. But these and other "lifestyle" changes have considerably less risk-reducing impact compared to prophylactic surgery.

4. All names for interviewees are pseudonyms.

5. The FORCE message boards include seventeen forums that range across a spectrum of broad and narrow topics (e.g., the "main forum," which includes posts on almost all aspects of HBOC versus "partner and spouse forum," which includes threads for those whose partner or spouse is dealing with HBOC). For this study, I sampled threads only from the main forum because it is the most commonly used (having over thirty thousand posts) and includes posts on the widest variety of issues, including medical practices related to BRCA risk. To sample a manageable number of threads, I focused on just one year, 2015. I read through the titles of all of the threads for that year, making a list of those that referenced any kind of medical practice associated with BRCA risk—not just screening practices but also practices associated with exercise, diet, surgery, hormonal therapy, anything that could be understood as a practice through which BRCA risk is enacted. (This meant excluding threads whose titles referenced things clearly not linked to medical practices, for instance, organizing support group meetings and debating developments in genetic research.) I cast my net wide at this stage of the research because I had not yet decided to focus only on screening practices. However, even when I did decide to narrow my focus to just screening practices, I was glad I had cast my net wide because threads that began with a question or concern about a non-screening-related practice, for instance, PBSO or chemoprevention, often included descriptions of screening practices. When I finished going through all the threads for 2015 on the main forum, I had a list of 244 threads whose titles referenced medical practices. This was too many to read (especially since each thread contained multiple, sometimes more than twenty-five, posts), so I numbered them and used a random number generator to reduce the list of threads to ninety-one. I then cut and pasted those threads into a Word document, excluding any identifying information, whether name, user name, or link, as per the restrictions of Virginia Tech IRB # 15–880. This yielded 137 pages of text to read.

6. High lifetime risk for breast cancer is considered to be 20 percent or greater. Interestingly, I never found an article, website, or guidebook that indicated what is considered high lifetime risk of ovarian cancer, but since the average lifetime risk is 1 to 2 percent, it stands to reason that anything over this is considered high.

7. Breast awareness (that is, knowing the feel of one's breasts well enough to notice significant changes) replaced breast self-exams in the 2009 NCCN guidelines due to research showing that the former had no impact on reducing breast cancer mortality.

8. As I explained in chapter 1, screening for ovarian cancer risk is not actually recommended by the NCCN. Their recommendation is PBSO by age thirty-five or forty. But if

BRCA+ women choose screening for ovarian cancer risk, these practices, pelvic exam, transvaginal ultrasound, and CA-125 testing, are the standard of care.

9. The idea that practices "do" or enact bodies is very much a praxiographic idea but not one that comes directly from *The Body Multiple*. Instead it comes from the subsequent 2004 essay by Mol and John Law, "Embodied Action, Enacted Bodies: The Example of Hypoglycemia." While Mol and Law's primary purpose in this essay is to explain how hypoglycemia is enacted in the daily lives of people with diabetes, they also ask how the condition "does" the diabetic body (45). In other words, they want to know what the body is "made to be" when enacted by hypoglycemia (50). What they find is that through all of the practices associated with hypoglycemia—eating, chewing, pricking, measuring, and so on—the diabetic body is enacted as a metabolic system, one in which "appreciating food is a matter of calculating carbohydrates and doing exercise is a way of burning sugar" (54). Other conditions can enact the body in a similar way, but the realities that result from those enactments are different. For instance, trying to lose weight also enacts the body as a metabolic system, but in this case "food consists of calories and physical exercise is a way to lose these" (54).

10. As I explained earlier, the 2016 NCCN guidelines for BRCA risk do not support screening for ovarian cancer on the basis that there is no data to support its effectiveness. See also Olivier et al.'s 2006 "CA-125 and Transvaginal Ultrasound Monitoring in High-Risk Women."

11. In the context of radiologic imaging, sensitivity refers to a test's ability to identify all instances of the condition, that is, to not produce any false negative results. Specificity refers to a test's ability to distinguish actual instances of the condition from those that might mimic it, that is, to not produce any false positive results.

12. The phrase "busy breasts" is a commonly used expression for describing dense, lumpy breasts that produce frequent findings (e.g., cysts and fibroadenomas) when examined or imaged. The idea that something could be "hiding" was expressed in a FORCE thread "How High a Risk to Justify a PBM?" The original contributor wrote: "I have heterogeneously dense breast tissue (not extremely dense). While I did have a lump that imaged as B-rads 5, it turned out to be nothing. It was a granular cell tumor (very rare, images just like BC [breast cancer], but has nothing to do with BC or BC risk, and not likely to recur). Of course, who the heck knows what is hiding in there that hasn't shown up on imaging or what could crop up in a short interval . . . that is where I worry, and that is what makes this screening situation so unbearable."

13. Like the message boards of other online support groups, the main forum of the FORCE boards includes more posts about abnormal or troubling screening results than normal ones. BRCA+ women are more likely to post, in other words, when a screening experience goes wrong than when it goes right. (Though often they will post to celebrate the news of a clean scan.) This fact would make me reluctant to use FORCE message board data if the medical literature, much of which I cite in this chapter, did not show that receiving abnormal screening results is *not* an anomaly for BRCA+ women.

14. Take, for example, the 2015 study, "Effects of False-Positive Cancer Screenings and Worry on Risk-Reducing Surgery Among BRCA1/2 Carriers." Here, authors David Portnoy, Jennifer Loud, and Paul Han argue that decisions to have risk-reducing surgery are influenced by several factors, "including an individual's objective cancer risk and her subjective perception of that risk" (710). What they call "perception of risk" is a key determinant of health-protective behaviors, but their point is that this perception is more complicated than we've thought insofar as it is affected more by emotional factors like worry and anxiety than cognitive ones (710). Focusing on the role that false positive test results might play in this perception, they argue that "increased rates and frequencies of screening may further heighten

the perceived cancer risk among BRCA mutation carriers because they serve as a repeated reminder of their high-risk status, further exacerbated by the unavoidable high frequency of screening test-related false-positive test results (FPTR)" (710). While their study did not show a strong association of FPTR with the decision to choose risk-reducing surgery, it did show that "the receipt of an FPTR was associated with changes in worry, and cancer worry was a strong predictor of surgical uptake in this high-risk population" (715).

15. For studies of the overestimation of breast cancer risk, see Black et al.'s "Perceptions of Breast Cancer Risk and Screening Effectiveness in Women Younger than 50 Years of Age" and Wang et al.'s "Comparison of Risk Perceptions and Beliefs Across Common Chronic Diseases."

16. In a FORCE thread called "Abnormal MRI—linear non mass enhancement," for example, a woman described her first experience with MRI as a "big roller coaster," explaining that its results led first to "an u/s guided biopsy, which was unsuccessful bcs it didn't show up on u/s, then an mri-guided biopsy, which was inconclusive, and finally a surgical biopsy." In the end and "after 6 weeks of stress," she reported, the findings were determined benign. Patricia Falls used similar terms to describe her experience with screening in "Waiting for Cancer," a 2016 op-ed published in the *New York Times*. The three years since getting a positive BRCA result, she wrote, "have featured a series of false alarms that take me on an emotional roller coaster. We are technologically ahead of the curve and diagnostically behind. Each six-month checkup for ovarian cancer is followed by a CA-125 blood test that delivers false-positive results, followed by a second a few weeks later that is normal. The MRIs, sonograms, and mammograms can detect potential malignancies with such great detail, but our ability to understand just what we're seeing hasn't caught up yet. Each and every mammogram or breast ultrasound in the last three years has been followed by additional tests after the detection of a 'suspicious area.' If the tests are negative, I will receive a note in the mail for another six-month follow-up, if they find something suspicious, I will receive a call from my doctor the next day. Inevitably, I get the call."

17. The BI-RADS assessment categories for breast MRI are 0 for incomplete findings, 1 for negative findings, 2 for benign findings, 3 for probably benign findings, 4 for suspicious findings, 5 for highly suspicious findings, and 6 for findings known through biopsy to be malignant (Morris et al. 137).

18. When surgical biopsies are image-guided, they are called "wire localization" biopsies because wires are placed in the area of the lesion during imaging (mammogram, MRI, or ultrasound) and then the patient is taken to an operating room where a surgeon uses the wire to identify the location of the lesion and then removes all or part of it.

Chapter 4

1. A good example of a text that uses topoi to both explain and change what is happening in a particular "substantive field" is Walsh and Prelli's "Getting Down in the Weeds to Get a God's-Eye View," their contribution to the 2017 collection, *Topologies as Techniques for a Post-Critical Rhetoric*. Here Walsh and Prelli explain how a synoptic topology composed of both visual and verbal topoi created a "view from nowhere" in early American discourses of ecology. This view helped to move ecology into "the stratosphere of the true sciences," but it did so at the expense of "the experiential ethos of others who engage directly with the resources in question" (210–11). Walsh and Prelli argue that synoptic topologies operate not just in ecological discourses but also in those of health and medicine, economics, and education, and that they can constrain those discourses in way that make "locality, situation, and subjectivity

appear to disappear" (210–11). While they warn critics to be on the look out for the operation of such topologies, they also suggest alternative topoi that might foster counterrhetorics, for instance the rhetoric of "biopiracy" that emerged from the "bioprospecting" topoi used by indigenous activists in defending the Amazonian rain forests against exploitation (211). This topic is also discussed by Leah Ceccarelli (but as a metaphor) in her 2013 *On the Frontier of Science*, a book I discuss in the concluding chapter.

2. "Hermeneutical rhetoric" is Michael Leff's term for understanding the inseparability between rhetoric and hermeneutics. Like Steven Mailloux, Leff wants to understand how hermeneutics relies on or employs rhetorical strategies, but he flips the terms, prioritizing the production of rhetoric (political rhetoric specifically) and asking how it employs or depends on hermeneutic strategies ("Hermeneutical Rhetoric" 198). But the point about their relationship is the same, namely that "we might say that all interpretive work involves participation in rhetorical exchange, and every rhetorical exchange involves some interpretive work" (198).

3. In post-process composition theory, this inseparability becomes more of an engulfment, as invention is completely absorbed into interpretation. Thomas Kent argues, for instance, that rhetoric has no truly heuristic or inventive function since each new "invention" is the product of the rhetor's interpretation of various situations, codes, and contexts. Writing is thus a kind of communicative interaction that is based entirely on "hermeneutic guesswork" and is not convention-bound, meaning that it cannot be codified in any meaningful way ("Paralogic Rhetoric" 145, 148).

4. Various 1960s and '70s arguments about the epistemic nature of rhetoric helped contribute to this reasoning, with many of them drawing on the work of New Rhetoric scholars like Kenneth Burke, Stephen Toulmin, and Chaim Perelman and Lucie Olbrechts-Tyteca. In his 1967 essay, "On Viewing Rhetoric as Epistemic," for instance, Robert Scott turned to Toulmin's distinction between analytic and substantial arguments in order to question belief in a priori truths, thus opening up more epistemic ground for rhetoric, which he understood as "not as a matter of giving effectiveness to truth but of creating it" (13).

5. See, for instance, Depew's "Revisiting Richard McKeon's Architectonic Rhetoric," the 2010 essay in which he explains McKeon's impact on the formation of rhetoric of science as a field of study, as well as the development of the Project on the Rhetoric of Inquiry (POROI) in the mid-1980s (49).

6. See Latour and Woolgar's *Laboratory Life*, particularly page 64 where they explain the function of inscription devices, arguing that the bioassay, for instance, "is not merely a means of obtaining some independently given entity; the bioassay constitutes the construction of the substance. Similarly a substance could not be said to exist without fractioning columns since a fraction exists only by virtue of the process of discrimination [. . .]. It is not simply that the phenomena depend on certain material instrumentation; rather the phenomena are thoroughly constituted by the material setting of the laboratory. The artificial reality, which participants describe in terms of an objective entity, has in fact been constructed by the use of inscription devices" (64).

7. Muckelbauer identifies McKeon's work as a key source for this move, arguing that in his effort to expand the scope of rhetoric, that is, to make it architectonic, McKeon helped to render rhetoric as indistinguishable from a practice of epistemological invention (20–21). "If the very production of truth and knowledge are subject to context and contingency," Muckelbauer writes, "then rhetoric becomes a generalized art of invention, an architectonic rubric for all modes of inquiry" (21). As a result of this development, rhetoric not only offers "a compatible conceptual milieu" for articulating an alternative to foundationalist epistemology "but almost seems to identify itself with that project," becoming "indistinguishable from

the massive, interdisciplinary effort to rethink the basic principles that engineer western conceptions of truth, knowledge, and inquiry" (25).

8. This idea of engaging texts or ideas not in order to know them but rather to do something different with them is illustrated well in Muckelbauer's discussion of situatedness and singularity in chapter 6 of *Future of Invention*. There, he argues against a "wealth of scholarship" showing that "rhetorical action is irreducible to reasoned principles or generalized methods," that "such principles and methods may well offer practices through which the capacity to be affected by actual situations can be provoked" (122). For example, even if we must acknowledge (as scholars like Thomas Kent have argued) that pedagogical tools like textbooks cannot accurately represent the processes of creating and analyzing discourse, "that need not mean that such textbooks should be abandoned or even revised. It might simply indicate that such textbooks do not function as representations (despite what any teacher or student might have said or thought); they might, rather, rather have functioned as singular provocations" (122).

9. See Pender, "Somatic Individuality in Context."

10. Such framing is common, for instance, in arguments that physicians and institutions need to supplement or balance the "medical model" of decision making and treatment with one that better accounts for patient perspective about quality of life. See, for instance, Asadi-Lari et al.'s "Patients' Needs, Satisfaction, and Health Related Quality of Life."

11. Hannah made this point when I interviewed her, arguing that feminist "lessons we've learned from breast cancer can't all be neatly mapped over BRCA." "While I think most people would prefer less invasive options," she continued, "it's infuriating to see people discuss PBM for BRCA+ women as though it's the same as mastectomy for BRCA- women, which happens all the time."

12. Dubriwny never explicitly claims that having room to question biomedicine will bring BRCA+ women real empowerment. Yet that is the implication of her argument. If the PBM narrative cannot fulfill its promise of empowerment because it portrays BRCA+ women as uncritical consumers of biomedical treatments and services, then it stands to reason that becoming (or being portrayed as) critical consumers will bring the opposite effect: real empowerment.

13. As Latour puts it in *Reassembling the Social*, contrary to what happens in the natural sciences, "the task of explaining" in the social sciences (and in the humanities, typically) "starts only after a profound *suspicion* has been introduced about the very existence of the object to be accounted for" (102; emphasis added).

Conclusion

1. For a thorough rebuttal of Young's understanding of romanticist notions of art, see Byron Hawk's *Counter-History of Composition*.

Bibliography

Abe, Hiroyuki, et al. "MR-Detected ('Second Look') Ultrasound Examination for Breast Lesions Detected Initially on MRI: MR and Sonographic Findings." *American Journal of Roentgenology*, vol. 194, 2009, pp. 370–77.

Alcorn, Marshall. *Changing the Subject in English Class: Discourse and the Constructions of Desires*. Southern Illinois UP, 2002.

Aristotle. *Nicomachean Ethics*. Translated by David Ross, Oxford UP, 1925.

———. *On Rhetoric: A Theory of Civic Discourse*. Translated by George A. Kennedy, Oxford UP, 2007.

Aronowitz, Robert. *Unnatural History: Breast Cancer and American Society*. Cambridge UP, 2007.

Asadi-Lari et al. "Patients' Needs, Satisfaction, and Health Related Quality of Life: Towards a Comprehensive Model." *Health and Quality of Life Outcomes*, vol. 2, no. 32, 2004, doi:10.1186/1477-7525-2-32. Accessed 17 June 2017.

Atwill, Janet. "Finding a Home or Making a Path." *Perspectives on Rhetorical Invention*, edited by Janet Atwill and Janice Lauer, U of Tennessee P, 2003.

———. *Rhetoric Reclaimed: Aristotle and the Liberal Arts Tradition*. Cornell UP, 1998.

Barnett, Scot. *Rhetorical Realism: Rhetoric, Ethics, and the Ontology of Things*. Routledge, 2016.

Barnett, Scot, and Casey Boyle, eds. *Rhetoric Through Everyday Things*. U of Alabama P, 2016.

Bennett, Jane. *Vibrant Matter: A Political Ecology of Things*. Duke UP, 2010.

Black, William C., et al. "Perceptions of Breast Cancer Risk and Screening Effectiveness in Women Younger than 50 Years of Age." *Journal of the National Cancer Institute*, vol. 87, no. 10, 1995, pp. 720–31.

Blake Scott, John. *Risky Rhetoric: AIDS and the Cultural Practices of HIV Testing*. Southern Illinois UP, 2003.

Boesky, Amy. *What We Have: One Family's Inspiring Story about Love, Loss, and Survival*. Gotham, 2010.

Bougie, O., and J. I. Weberpals. "Clinical Considerations of BRCA1- and BRCA2-Mutation Carriers: A Review." *International Journal of Surgical Oncology*, vol. 2011, 2011, pp. 1–11.

Bradbury, A. R., et al. "Uptake and Timing of Bilateral Salpingo-Oophorectomy Among BRCA1 and BRCA2 Mutation Carriers." *Genetics in Medicine*, vol. 10, no. 3, 2008, pp. 161–66.

"Breast Magnetic Resonance Imaging (MRI)." *Johns Hopkins Medicine Health Library*, https://www.Hopkinsmedicine.org/healthlibrary/test_procedures/gynecology /breast_magnetic_resonance_imaging_mri_92,P09110/. Accessed 22 June 2016.

Bryant, Levi. *The Democracy of Objects*. MPublishing, 2011.

Bueger, Christian. "Pathways to Practice: Praxiography and International Politics." *European Political Science Review*, vol. 6, no. 3, 2013, pp. 383–406.

Bunton, Robin. "Popular Health, Advanced Liberalism, and *Good Housekeeping* Magazine." *Foucault, Health, and Medicine*, edited by Alan Petersen and Robin Bunton, Routledge, 1997, pp. 223–48.

Bunton, Robin, and Alan Petersen, eds. *Genetic Governance: Health, Risk, and Ethics in the Biotech Era.* Routledge, 2005.

Burchell, Graham, et al., eds. *The Foucault Effect: Studies in Governmentality.* U of Chicago P, 1991.

Burke, Kenneth. "What Are the Signs of What?" *Anthropological Linguistics,* vol. 4, no. 6, 1962, pp. 1–23.

Castel, Robert. "From Dangerousness to Risk." Burchell et al., pp. 281–98.

Ceccarelli, Leah. *On the Frontier of Science: An American Rhetoric of Exploration and Exploitation.* Michigan State UP, 2013.

Chandler, Daniel. *Semiotics: The Basics.* Routledge, 2002.

Chen, S., and G. Parmigiani. "Meta-Analysis of BRCA1 and BRCA2 Penetrance." *Journal of Clinical Oncology,* vol. 25, no. 11, 2007, pp. 1329–33.

Chopier, J., et al. "Radiopathological Correlations: Masses, Non-Masslike Enhancements, And MRI-Guided Biopsy." *Diagnostic and Interventional Imaging* 95, 2014, pp. 213–25.

Condit, Celeste. "The Materiality of Coding: Rhetoric, Genetics, and the Matter of Life." *Rhetorical Bodies,* edited by Jack Selzer and Sharon Crowley, U of Wisconsin P, 1999, pp. 326–56.

———. *The Meanings of the Gene: Public Debates About Human Heredity.* U of Wisconsin P, 1999.

Coole, Diana, and Samantha Frost, eds. *New Materialisms: Ontology, Agency, and Politics.* Duke UP, 2010.

Couch, Fergus, et al. "Two Decades After BRCA: Setting Paradigms in Personalized Cancer Care and Prevention." *Science* 343, 2014, pp. 1466–69.

Crabb, Shona, and Amanda LeCouteur. "'Fiona Farewells Her Breasts': A Popular Magazine Account of Breast Cancer Prevention." *Critical Public Health,* vol. 16, no. 1, 2006, pp. 5–18.

Dall, Barbara J. G., et al. "Reporting and Management of Breast Lesions Detected Using MRI." *Clinical Radiology,* vol. 66, no. 12, 2011, pp. 1120–28.

Davies, Kevin, and Michael White. *Breakthrough: The Race to Find the Breast Cancer Gene.* Wiley, 1996.

Dean, Mitchell. *Governmentality: Power and Rule in Modern Society.* Sage, 1999.

Decoding Annie Parker. Directed by Steven Bernstein. Entertainment One Films, 2013.

Dent, Rebecca, and Ellen Warner. "Screening for Hereditary Breast Cancer." *Seminars in Oncology,* vol. 34, no. 5, 2007, pp. 392–400.

Depew, David. "Revisiting Richard McKeon's Architectonic Rhetoric: A Response to 'The Uses of Rhetoric in a Technological Age: Architectonic Productive Arts.'" *Reengaging the Prospects of Rhetoric,* edited by Mark J. Porovecchio, Routledge, 2010, pp. 37–56.

Diedrich, Lisa, and Emily Boyce. "'Breast Cancer on Long Island': The Emergence of a New Object Through Mapping Practices." *Biosocieties,* vol. 2, no. 2, 2007, pp. 193–218.

Dubriwny, Tasha N. *The Vulnerable Empowered Woman: Feminism, Postfeminism, and Women's Health.* Rutgers UP, 2013.

Duster, Troy. *Backdoor to Eugenics.* Routledge, 1990.

Eberly, Rosa A. *Citizen Critics: Literary Public Spheres.* U of Illinois P, 2000.

Eby, Peter R., et al. "Probably Benign Lesions Detected on Breast MR Imaging." *Magnetic Resonance Imaging Clinics,* vol. 18, no. 2, 2010, pp. 309–21.

Eby, Peter R., et al. "Characteristics of Probably Benign Breast MRI Lesions." *American Journal of Roentgenology,* vol. 193, no. 3, 2009, pp. 861–67.

Ewald, François. "Insurance and Risk." Burchell et al., pp. 197–210.

Fahnestock, Jeanne, and Marie Secor. "The Rhetoric of Literary Criticism." *Textual Dynamics of the Profession: Historical and Contemporary Studies of Writing in Professional Com-*

munities, edited by Charles Bazerman and James Paradis, U of Wisconsin P, 1991, pp. 76–96.

Falls, Patricia. "Op-Ed: Waiting for Cancer." *New York Times*, 1 Sept. 2016.

Felski, Rita. *The Limits of Critique*. U of Chicago P, 2015.

Foucault, Michel. "Governmentality." Burchell et al., pp. 87–104.

Friedman, Sue, et al. *Confronting Hereditary Breast and Ovarian Cancer: Identify Your Risk, Understand Your Options, Change Your Destiny*. Johns Hopkins UP, 2012.

Gaonkar, Dilip. "The Idea of Rhetoric in the Rhetoric of Science." *Rhetorical Hermeneutics: Invention and Interpretation in the Age of Science*, edited by Alan Gross, State U of New York P, 1997, pp. 25–88.

Gessen, Masha. *Blood Matters: From Inherited Illness to Designer Babies, How the World and I Found Ourselves in the Future of the Gene*. Harvest Books, 2009.

Graham, S. Scott. "Object-Oriented Ontology's Binary Duplication and the Promise of Thing-Oriented Ontologies." *Rhetoric Through Everyday Things*, edited by Scot Barnett and Casey Boyle, U of Alabama P, 2016, pp. 108–22.

———. *The Politics of Pain Medicine: A Rhetorical-Ontological Inquiry*. U of Chicago P, 2015.

Graham, S. Scott, and Carl Herndl. "Multiple Ontologies in Pain Management: Toward a Postplural Rhetoric of Science." *Technical Communication Quarterly*, vol. 22, no. 2, 2013, pp. 103–25.

Greene, Ronald Walter. "Another Materialist Rhetoric." *Critical Studies in Mass Communication* 15, 1998, pp. 21–40.

———. "Rhetorical Materialism: The Rhetorical Subject and the General Intellect." *Rhetoric, Materiality, and Politics*, edited by Barbara A. Biesecker and John L. Lucaites, Peter Lang, 2009, pp. 43–65.

Gronnvoll, Marita, and Jamie Landau. "From Viruses to Russian Roulette to Dance: A Rhetorical Critique and Creation of Genetic Metaphors." *Rhetoric Society Quarterly*, vol. 40, no. 1, 2010, pp. 46–70.

Gross, Alan. "The Origin of the Species: Evolutionary Taxonomy as an Example of the Rhetoric of Science." *The Rhetorical Turn: Invention and Persuasion in the Conduct of Inquiry*, edited by Herbert W. Simons, U of Chicago P, 1990, pp. 91–115.

———. *The Rhetoric of Science*. Harvard UP, 1996.

———. *Starring the Text: The Place of Rhetoric in Science Studies*. Southern Illinois UP, 2006.

Hallowell, Nina. "Doing the Right Thing: Genetic Risk and Responsibility." *Sociology of Health and Illness*, vol. 21, no. 5, 1999, pp. 597–621.

Happe, Kelly E. *The Material Gene: Gender, Race, and Heredity After the Human Genome Project*. New York UP, 2013.

Harman, Graham. *Prince of Networks: Bruno Latour and Metaphysics*. re.press, 2009.

———. *Towards Speculative Realism: Essays and Lectures*. Zero Books, 2010.

Hasain, Marouf A. *The Rhetoric of Eugenics in Anglo-American Thought*. U of Georgia P, 1996.

Hauser, Gerard, and Donald P. Cushman. "McKeon's Philosophy of Communication: The Architectonic and Interdisciplinary Arts." *Philosophy and Rhetoric*, vol. 6, no. 4, 1973, pp. 211–34.

Hawk, Byron. *A Counter-History of Composition: Toward Methodologies of Complexity*. U of Pittsburgh P, 2007.

"Health-Related Quality of Life and Well-Being." *Office of Disease Prevention and Health Promotion*, http://www.healthypeople.gov/2020/about/foundation-health-measures /Health-Related-Quality-of-Life-and-Well-Being. Accessed 15 Sept. 2016.

Hedgecoe, Adam. "Ethical Boundary Work: Geneticization, Philosophy, and the Social Sciences." *Medicine, Health Care, and Philosophy*, vol. 4, no. 3, 2001, pp. 305–9.

————. "Reconstructing Geneticization: A Research Manifesto." *Health Law Journal* 7, 1999, pp. 5–18.

Hoedemaekers, Rogeer, and Henk ten Have. "Geneticization: The Cyprus Paradigm." *Journal of Medicine and Philosophy*, vol. 23, no. 3, 1998, pp. 247–87.

Hollowell, Lauren, et al. "Lesion Morphology on Breast MRI Affects Targeted Ultrasound Correlation Rate." *European Journal of Radiology*, vol. 25, no. 5, 2015, pp. 1279–84.

Hubbard, Ruth, and Elijah Wald. *Exploding the Gene Myth: How Genetic Information Is Produced and Manipulated by Scientists, Physicians, Employers, Insurance Companies, Educators, and Law Enforcers.* Beacon Press, 1993.

Illich, Ivan. *Medical Nemesis: The Expropriation of Health.* Pantheon, 1976.

In the Family. Directed by Joanna Rudnick. Viacom Media Networks, 2008.

Johansen, Jorgen Dines, and Svend Erik Larsen. *Signs in Use: An Introduction to Semiotics.* Routledge, 2002.

Jolie, Angelina. "Op-Ed: Diary of a Surgery." *New York Times*, 24 March 2015, A23.

————. "Op-Ed: My Medical Choice." *New York Times*, 14 May 2013, A25.

Kent, Thomas. *Paralogic Rhetoric: A Theory of Communicative Interaction.* Bucknell UP, 1993.

Keranen, Lisa. "Conspectus: Inventing Futures for the Rhetoric of Science, Technology, and Medicine." *POROI: An International Journal of Rhetorical Analysis and Invention*, vol. 9, no. 1, 2013, doi:10.13008/2151–2957.1167. Accessed 3 Mar. 2014.

Kerr, Anne, et al. "Eugenics and the New Genetics in Britain: Examining Contemporary Professionals' Accounts." *Science, Technology, and Human Values*, vol. 23, no. 2, 1998, pp. 175–99.

Klawiter, Maren. *The Biopolitics of Breast Cancer: Changing Cultures of Disease and Activism.* Minneapolis: U of Minnesota P, 2008.

Kupfer, Fern. *Leaving Long Island . . . and Other Departures.* Lulu, 2012.

Latour, Bruno. "An Attempt at a 'Compositionist Manifesto.'" *New Literary History*, vol. 41, no. 3, 2010, pp. 471–90.

————. *Reassembling the Social: An Introduction to Actor-Network Theory.* Oxford UP, 2007.

————. *We Have Never Been Modern.* Translated by Catherine Porter, Harvard UP, 1993.

————. "Why Has Critique Run Out of Steam? From Matters of Fact to Matters of Concern." *Critical Inquiry*, vol. 30, 2004, pp. 225–48.

Latour, Bruno, and Steven Woolgar. *Laboratory Life: The Construction of Scientific Facts.* Princeton UP, 1986.

Law, John. *After Method: Mess in Social Science Research.* Routledge, 2004.

————. "Enacting Naturecultures: A View from STS." 2004. heterogeneities.net/publications/Law2004EnactingNaturecultures.pdf.

Law, John, and Vicky Singleton. "Object Lessons." *Organization*, vol. 12, no. 3, 2005, pp. 331–55.

Leff, Michael. "Hermeneutical Rhetoric." *Rhetoric and Hermeneutics in Our Time*, edited by Walter Jost and Michael J. Hyde, Yale UP, 1997, pp. 196–214.

————. "The Topics of Argumentative Invention in Latin Rhetorical Theory from Cicero to Boethius." *Rhetorica*, vol. 1, no. 1, 1983, pp. 23–44.

Lehman, Constance D., and Robert A. Smith. "The Role of MRI in Breast Cancer Screening." *Journal of the National Comprehensive Cancer Network*, vol. 7, no. 10, 2009, pp. 1109–15.

Lemke, Thomas. *Foucault, Governmentality, and Critique.* Paradigm Publishers, 2011.

Lerner, Barron H. *The Breast Cancer Wars: Fear, Hope, and the Pursuit of a Cure in Twentieth-Century America.* Oxford UP, 2003.

Leung, Jessica. "Second-Look Ultrasound: Only for Biopsy or More?" *European Journal of Radiology*, vol. 81, no. 1, 2012, pp. S87–S89.

————. "Utility of Second-Look Ultrasound in the Evaluation of MRI-Detected Breast Lesions." *Seminars in Roentgenology*, vol. 46, no. 4, 2011, pp. 260–74.

Lewontin, R. C. *Biology as Ideology: The Doctrine of DNA.* Harper Perennial, 1992.

Lewontin, R. C., et al. *Not in Our Genes: Biology, Ideology, and Human Nature.* Pantheon Books, 1984.

Liberman, Laura, et al. "Probably Benign Lesions at Breast Magnetic Resonance Imaging: Preliminary Experience in High-Risk Women." *Cancer*, vol. 98, no. 2, 2003, pp. 377–88.

Lippman, Abby. "The Politics of Health: Geneticization Versus Health Promotion." *The Politics of Women's Health*, edited by Susan Sherwin, Temple UP, 1998, pp. 64–82.

————. "Prenatal Testing and Screening: Constructing Needs and Reinforcing Inequalities." *American Journal of Law and Medicine*, vol. 17, 1991, pp. 15–50.

Lock, Margaret. "Breast Cancer: Reading the Omens." *Anthropology*, vol. 14, no. 4, 1998, pp. 7–16.

Lorde, Audre. *The Cancer Journals.* Aunt Lute Books, 1980.

Lourenco, Ana P., et al. "Utility of Targeted Sonography in Management of Probably Benign Lesions Identified on Magnetic Resonance Imaging." *Journal of Ultrasound Medicine*, vol. 31, 2012, pp. 1033–40.

Lupton, Deborah. *The Imperative of Health: Public Health and the Regulated Body.* Sage, 1995.

————. *Risk and Sociocultural Theory: New Directions and Perspectives.* Cambridge UP, 2000.

————. "Risk as Moral Danger: The Social and Political Functions of Risk Discourse in Public Health." *International Journal of Health Services*, vol. 23, no. 3, 1993, pp. 425–35.

Mahoney, Mary C., and Mary S. Newell. "Breast Intervention: How I Do It." *Radiology*, vol. 268, no. 1, 2013, pp. 12–24.

Mailloux, Steven. "Articulation and Understanding: The Pragmatic Intimacy Between Rhetoric and Hermeneutics." *Rhetoric and Hermeneutics in Our Time*, edited by Walter Jost and Michael J. Hyde, Yale UP, 1997, pp. 378–94.

Mak, Geertje. *Doubting Sex: Inscriptions, Bodies, and Selves in Nineteenth-Century Hermaphrodite Case Histories.* Manchester UP, 2013.

Marback, Richard. "Unclenching the Fist: Embodying Rhetoric and Giving Objects Their Due." *Rhetoric Society Quarterly*, vol. 38, no. 1, 2008, pp. 46–65.

Marx, Karl. *Capital.* Translated by Ben Fowkes, vol. 2, Vintage, 1977.

McKeon, Richard. "The Uses of Rhetoric in a Technological Age: Architectonic Productive Arts." *Rhetoric: Essays in Invention and Discovery*, edited by Mark Backman, Ox Bow Press, 1987, pp. 1–24.

Miller, Carolyn. "The Aristotelian *Topos*: Hunting for Novelty." *Rereading Aristotle's Rhetoric*, edited by Alan Gross and Arthur E. Walzer, Southern Illinois UP, 2008, pp. 130–46.

Miller, Carolyn, and Jack Selzer. "Special Topics of Argument in Engineering Reports." *Writing in Non-Academic Settings*, edited by Lee Odell and Dixie Goswami, Guilford, 1985, pp. 309–41.

Mol, Annemarie. *The Body Multiple: Ontology in Medical Practice.* Duke UP, 2004.

————. *The Logic of Care: Health and the Problem of Patient Choice.* Routledge, 2008.

————. "Missing Links, Making Links: The Performance of Some Atheroscleroses." *Differences in Medicine: Unraveling Practices, Techniques and Bodies*, edited by Marc Berg and Annemarie Mol, Duke UP, 1998, pp. 144–65.

————. "Ontological Politics: A Word and Some Questions." *Actor Network Theory and After*, edited by John Law and John Hassard, Blackwell Publishing, 1999, pp. 74–89.

————. "Proving or Improving: On Health Care Research as a Form of Self-Reflection." *Qualitative Health Research*, vol. 16, no. 3, 2006, pp. 405–14.

Mol, Annemarie, and John Law. "Embodied Action, Enacted Bodies: The Example of Hypoglycemia." *Body and Society*, vol. 10, nos. 2–3, 2004, pp. 43–62.

Morris, E. A., et al. "ACR BI-RADS®: Magnetic Resonance Imaging." *ACR BI-RADS®* Atlas,
2013. https://www.acr.org/-/media/ACR/Files/RADS/BI-RADS/BIRADS-Poster
.pdf.

Morris, Joi L., and Ora K. Gordon. *Positive Results: Making the Best Decisions When You're at
High Risk for Breast or Ovarian Cancer*. Prometheus Books, 2010.

Muckelbauer, John. *The Future of Invention: Rhetoric, Postmodernism, and the Problem of
Change*. State U of New York P, 2008.

———. "On Reading Differently: Through Foucault's Resistance." *College English*, vol. 63, no.
1, 2000, pp. 71–94.

"NCCN Guidelines Version 2.2017 BRCA-Related Breast and/or Ovarian Cancer
Syndrome." National Comprehensive Cancer Network, http://www.nccn.org/pro
fessionals/physician_gls/PDF/genetics_screening.pdf. Accessed 22 June 2017.

Nelkin, Dorothy, and Susan Lindee. *The DNA Mystique: The Gene as Cultural Icon*. Freeman,
1995.

Nettleton, Sarah. "Governing the Risky Self: How to Become Happy, Healthy, and Wise."
Petersen and Bunton, 207–22.

Olivier, R. I., et al. "CA-125 and Transvaginal Ultrasound Monitoring in High-Risk Women
Cannot Prevent the Diagnosis of Advanced Ovarian Cancer." *Gynecologic Oncology*,
vol. 100, no. 1, 2006, pp. 20–26.

Pender, Kelly. "Genetic Subjectivity *in situ*: A Rhetorical Reading of Genetic Determinism
and Genetic Opportunity in the Biosocial Community of FORCE." *Rhetoric and
Public Affairs*, vol. 15, no. 2, 2012, pp. 319–49.

———. "Somatic Individuality in Context, a Comparative Case Study." *Public Understanding
of Science*, 2016. https://doi.org/10.1177/0963662516678116.

Petersen, Alan. "Facilitating Autonomy: The Discourse of Genetic Counseling." Petersen and
Bunton, *New Genetics*, pp. 135–58.

———. "Governmentality, Critical Scholarship, and the Medical Humanities." *Journal of
Medical Humanities*, vol. 24, 2003, pp. 187–201.

———. "The New Genetics and the Politics of Public Health." *Critical Public Health*, vol. 8,
1998, pp. 59–71.

———. "Risk and the Regulated Self: The Discourse of Health Promotion as Politics of
Uncertainty." *Journal of Sociology*, vol. 32, no. 1, 1996, pp. 44–57.

———. "The Scope and Context of the New Genetics." Petersen and Bunton, *New Genetics*,
pp. 35–66.

Petersen, Alan, and Robin Bunton, eds. *Foucault: Health and Medicine*. Routledge, 1997.

———. *The New Genetics and the Public's Health*. Routledge, 2002.

Petrucelli, Nancie, et al. "BRCA1- and BRCA2-Associated Hereditary Breast and Ovarian
Cancer." *Gene Reviews*, 2016, http://www.ncbi.nlm.nih.gov/books/NBK1247/.
Accessed 22 June 2017.

Plevritis, Sylvia, et al. "Cost-Effectiveness of Screening BRCA1/2 Mutation Carriers with
Breast Magnetic Resonance Imaging." *JAMA*, vol. 295, no. 20, 2006, pp. 2374–84.

Pollock, Jondavid and James S. Welsh. "Clinical Cancer Genetics Part 2: Breast." *American
Journal of Clinical Oncology*, vol. 37, no. 1, 2014, pp. 86–89.

Port, Diana R. *Previvors: Facing the Breast Cancer Gene and Making Life-Changing Decisions*.
Avery, 2010.

Portnoy, David, et al. "Effects of False-Positive Cancer Screenings and Worry on Risk-Reducing Surgery Among BRCA1/2 Carriers." *Health Psychology*, vol. 34, no. 7, 2015, pp. 709–17.

Prelli, Lawrence. *A Rhetoric of Science: Inventing Scientific Discourse*. U of South Carolina P, 1989.

Press, N., et al. "Collective Fear, Individualized Risk: The Social and Cultural Context of Genetic Testing for Breast Cancer." *Nursing Ethics*, vol. 7, no. 3, 2000, pp. 237–49.

Pullman, George. "Rhetoric and Hermeneutics: Composition, Invention, and Literature." *The Kinneavy Papers: Theory and the Study of Discourse*, edited by Lynn Worsham, Sidney Dobrin, and Gary Olsen, State U of New York P, 2000, pp. 155–82.

Queller, Jessica. *Pretty Is What Changes: Impossible Choices, the Breast Cancer Gene, and How I Defined My Destiny*. Spiegel & Grau, 2009.

Rabinow, Paul. "Artificiality and Enlightenment: From Sociobiology to Biosociality." *Incorporations*, edited by Jonathan Crary and Sanford Kwinter, Zone Books, 1992, pp. 234–52.

Raikhlin, Antony, et al. "Breast MRI as an Adjunct to Mammography for Breast Cancer Screening in High-Risk Patients: Retrospective Review." *American Journal of Roentgenology*, vol. 204, 2015, pp. 889–97.

Reckwitz, Andreas. "The Status of the 'Material' in Theories of Culture: From 'Social Structure' to 'Artefacts.'" *Journal for the Theory of Social Behaviour*, vol. 32, no. 2, 2002, pp. 195–217.

Rice, Jenny. *Distant Publics: Development Rhetoric and the Subject of Crisis*. U of Pittsburgh P, 2012.

Rickert, Thomas. *Acts of Enjoyment: Rhetoric, Zizek, and the Return of the Subject*. U of Pittsburgh P, 2007.

———. *Ambient Rhetoric: The Rhetorical Attunements of Being*. U of Pittsburgh P, 2013.

Robertson, Ann. "Embodying Risk, Embodying Political Rationality: Women's Accounts of Risks for Breast Cancer." *Health, Risk, and Society*, vol. 2, no. 2, 2000, pp. 220–35.

Rose, Nikolas. *The Politics of Life Itself: Biomedicine, Power, and Subjectivity in the Twenty-First Century*. U of Princeton P, 2007.

Rose, Nikolas, et al. "Governmentality." *Annual Review of Law and Social Science*, vol. 2, 2006, pp. 83–104.

Rylands-Monk, Frances. "BI-RADS 3 Lesions Prove Controversial and Pose Management Challenges." *European Congress of Radiology Today*, March 14, 2011, 13.

Sabatinos, Sarah A. "Replication Fork Stalling and the Fork Protection Complex." *Nature Education*, vol. 3, no. 9, 2010, p. 40.

Saslow, Debbie, et al. "American Cancer Society Guidelines for Breast Screening with MRI as an Adjunct to Mammography." *CA: A Cancer Journal for Clinicians*, vol. 57, no. 2, 2007, pp. 75–89.

Sauer, Beverly. *The Rhetoric of Risk: Technical Documentation in Hazardous Environments*. Routledge, 2003.

Scott, Blake, et al. "The Rhetorics of Health and Medicine: Inventional Possibilities for Scholarship and Engaged Practice." *POROI: An International Journal of Rhetorical Analysis and Invention*, vol. 9, no. 1, 2013.

Scott, Robert. "On Viewing Rhetoric as Epistemic." *Central States Speech Journal*, vol. 18, 1967, pp. 9–17.

Seigel, Marika. *The Rhetoric of Pregnancy*. U of Chicago P, 2013.

Simons, Herbert. "The Rhetoric of Inquiry as an Intellectual Movement." *The Rhetorical Turn: Invention and Persuasion in the Conduct of Inquiry*, edited by Herbert Simons, U of Chicago P, 1990, pp. 1–34.

Sloterdijk, Peter. *Critique of Cynical Reason*. U of Minnesota P, 1988.

Stark, Lizzie. *Pandora's DNA: Tracing the Breast Cancer Genes Through History, Science, and One Family Tree*. Chicago Review Press, 2014.

Sulik, Gayle. *Pink Ribbon Blues: How Breast Cancer Culture Undermines Women's Health*. Oxford UP, 2012.

"Survival Rates for Ovarian Cancer, by Stage." *American Cancer Society*, http://www.cancer .org/cancer/ovarian-cancer/detection-diagnosis-staging/survival-rates.html. Accessed 22 June 2017.

Ten Have, Henk. "Genetics and Culture: The Geneticization Thesis." *Medicine, Health Care, and Philosophy*, vol. 4, 2001, pp. 295–304.

Van Dijck, Jose. *Imagenation: Popular Images of Genetics*. New York UP, 1998.

Venkitaraman, A. R. "Cancer Suppression by the Chromosome Custodians, BRCA1 And BRCA2." *Science*, vol. 343, 2014, pp. 1470–75.

Vitanza, Victor. "'The Wasteland Grows'; Or, What is 'Cultural Studies for Composition' and Why Must We Always Speak Good of It?: ParaResponse to Julie Drew." *JAC*, vol. 19, no. 4, 1999, pp. 699–703.

Walsh, Lynda. "The Common Topoi of STEM Discourse: An Apologia and Methodological Proposal, with Pilot Survey." *Written Communication*, vol. 27, no. 1, 2010, pp. 120–56.

Walsh, Lynda, and Casey Boyle. *Topologies as Techniques for a Post-Critical Rhetoric*. Palgrave Macmillan, 2017.

Walsh, Lynda, and Lawrence J. Prelli. "Getting Down in the Weeds to Get a God's-Eye View: The Synoptic Topology of Early American Ecology." *Topologies as Techniques for a Post-Critical Rhetoric*, edited by Lynda Walsh and Casey Boyle, Palgrave Macmillan, 2017, pp. 197–218.

Wang, Catherine, et al. "Comparison of Risk Perceptions and Beliefs Across Common Chronic Diseases." *Preventive Medicine*, vol. 48, no. 2, 2009, pp. 197–202.

Wilder, Laura. *Rhetorical Strategies and Genre Conventions in Literary Studies: Teaching and Writing in the Disciplines*. Southern Illinois UP, 2012.

Woodward, E. R., et al. "Annual Surveillance by CA125 and Transvaginal Ultrasound for Ovarian Cancer in Both High-Risk and Population Risk Women Is Ineffective." *BJOG*, vol. 114, no. 12, 2007, pp. 1500–1509.

Woolgar, Steve, and Dorothy Pawluch. "Ontological Gerrymandering: The Anatomy of Social Problems Explanations." *Social Problems*, vol. 32, no. 3, 1985, pp. 214–27.

Young, Richard. "Arts, Crafts, Gifts, and Knacks: Some Disharmonies in the New Rhetoric." *Reinventing the Rhetorical Tradition*, edited by Ian Pringle and Avia Freedman, L and S Books, 1980, pp. 53–60.

Index